Prismatica

Prismatica

Long live the people!!

Claudia Chaney

Writers Club Press

San Jose New York Lincoln Shanghai

Prismatica
Long live the people!!

Writers Club Press
an imprint of iUniverse.com, Inc.

For information address:
iUniverse.com, Inc.
5220 S 16th, Ste. 200
Lincoln, NE 68512
www.iuniverse.com

ISBN: 0-595-18326-3

Printed in the United States of America

DEDICATION TO MY NANA, WHOM I WAS NAMED AFTER

Everyone has something to give…knowledge…a talent. When you use that talent to help others, everyone benefits. The following poems were handed down from Nana, to Grandmother, and now to me. I am not sure as to where they originally came from, or who wrote them. It could have been Nana, but I am not positive.

The Gift of Giving
The more you give, the more you get
The more you laugh, the less you fret
The more you do unselfishly, the more you'll live abundantly
The more of everything you share, the more you'll always have to spare
The more you love, the more you'll find…
That life is good, and friends are kind
For only what we give away, will enrich us every day.

Here's another one she always used to tell her kids
Be careful of the words you speak, and keep them soft and sweet
For you never know from time to time, which ones you'll have to eat.

To my family…Brooklynne, Hannah, John, Mom, Gramma and for all of those who truly care about living life to the fullest!

Contents

Section 1:
Physical necessities

WATER SOURCES

Water is a very important factor in physical health. It hydrates, and helps keep nutrients and energy flowing freely through the body. Water helps give shape to the cells, regulate body temperature, lubricate joints, and cushion body organs. Ordinarily, a good rule of thumb is to drink about 8 oz of water per day. Even a lack of only 2 oz per day, can leave you with 30% less energy than what you could have, by only drinking 2 oz. more. When waking up, one should drink not ice or cold water, but water at room temperature…something like hot tonic tea would be one of the best solutions for waking up in the morning. Something stimulating, but not addictive. The colder water is upon entering the system, the more energy is needed to warm the water to body temperature.

Holding Tank/Cistern

Catching rainwater on rooftops, and directing water into holding tanks (cisterns) has been the most common way of providing water to communities with little or no access to springs, or all—year—around fresh water streams, since before First Century BC. Even now, we rely on very similar methods. Look up on a hill in your area, or near a town; you'll see a holding tank, *above* the city, which contains the area's water supply. The only difference between those systems and a cistern is:

■ Of course their tanks are huge, in comparison to what you would need, even for a family of 20!

- They don't catch fresh water from the sky; they only hold water taken from the earth.
- The water they do hold has probably been recycled from sewage, ground water polluted with pesticides, etc. (Massive amounts of chlorine, and other potent chemicals to kill viruses, bacteria, and the like).

You can build a cistern, which is fed by fresh water streams, springs, and/or wells, if these resources are available to you. But if you don't have access to these sources of water, a combination of a rooftop, and/or a cistern to catch and hold water, is a perfect solution for someone with dry land!

Water Cistern

First, decide where you want your cistern to be; make sure the site you choose is at least 100 feet or more *above* where your house is (or will be).

Have someone hold the end of a rope/string at the center of where your cistern will be built. Follow the string or rope out several feet, or half the distance of what size you will want your cistern. Walk in a circle all the way around your helper, leaving a trail of flour behind you as you go. This will give you an idea as to where to dig your foundation.

Next, Dig a hole for the foundation; build the foundation the same as you would for your house. (Refer to Shelter chapter). Once you have finished the foundation, build a rock wall, about 10 feet tall, surrounding the foundation. (You don't need to dig a very big hole in the ground for the foundation; just berm the outsides of the wall with earth, as the wall ascends. You will want plenty of pressure coming from all outsides of the cistern to keep the wall from collapsing when it is filled with water). Leave a hole for water to exit from, close to the bottom of the cistern, and for any other entrances/exits to the cistern itself. Make the entrance/exit holes about ¼" larger than what your plumbing/pipes will be; once the pipes are connected from the larger to the smaller ones, this will help pressurize the system.

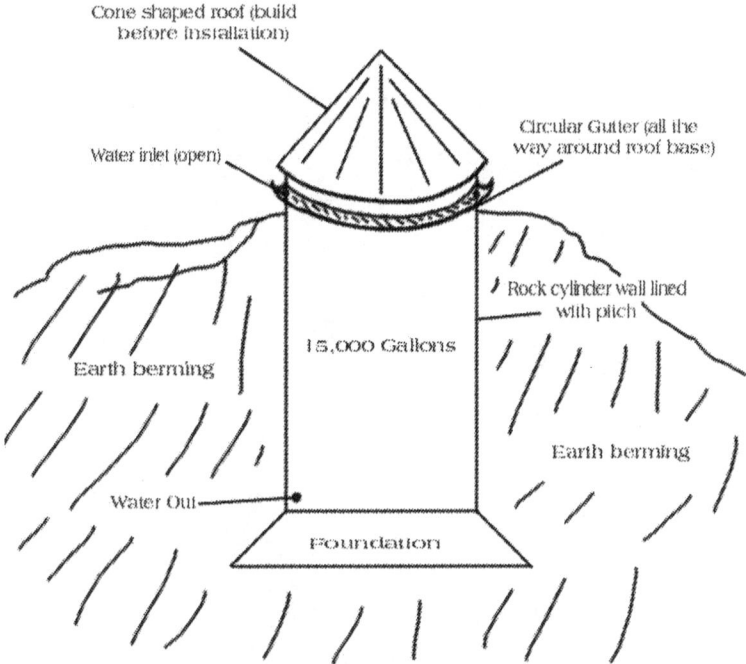

Seal all entrances and exits before and after installing the pipes. (Seal the interior and exterior of the walls, and roof as they are being built).

Build the roof in a similar manner as the one for your house; only shape it in the form of a cone. Attach a gutter all the way around the bottom of the structure, (right at the base of the roof), with one opening on each side of the cistern, (opposite of one another), which will lead into the cistern. Cover this gutter with ¼ or 1/8 inch wire mesh screen, to keep out debris. Clean the gutter out when necessary. Cover the feeding tubes with even finer screen. Clean these out as well, whenever necessary. The picture above graphically represents this design. (Sorry, I'm not much of an artist). The water inlets at the base of the roof allow the water from the gutters to go into the cistern, and help keep it from exploding from excess water pressure. Having the roof on top not only keeps out debris, but also keeps the water from evaporating with the heat of summer days.

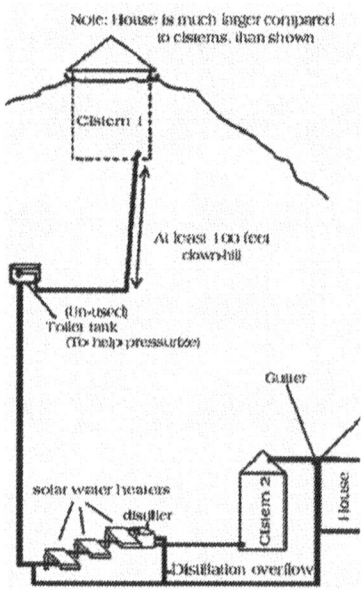

This picture shows a general idea as to what the cistern would look like, and where it should be, in relation to the house, distiller, solar water heaters, and the basic overall system.

In case you don't have property of your own, or are in need of immediate survival, look for patches of *coniferous* trees, bushes, or other leaf—bearing plants, among pine, juniper, or other plants that do not require a lot of water. If there is a spot that doesn't seem to venture along a path, there is most likely a spring present. If the coniferous foliage tends to follow a path, leading down a valley, it is probably a creek. Water, as does most everything else on this planet, follows the rule of gravity; it always goes down, as low as it can. Even if you do not see the water, dig a little (or a lot). You'll find it.

Creeks

Use some creeks for irrigation; you can make man—made creeks leading to the cistern for indoor use. To build your own creek, you need to find a spot to start from, which is of course at the highest elevation possible. Then, you just basically dig a ditch the width and depth you want it to be, and line it with rocks so the water isn't lost by being soaked up in the ground. If the water hasn't first gone through your purification system, and you are unsure of how pure the water is, boil the water first, if you plan on drinking it. If you are just using the creeks for irrigation, you can lead them to the orchard/s or gardens where you need them.

Irrigation

For all of the plants that require rich, moist, well—drained soil, plant them along little trenches (irrigation creeks), on a hillside facing SE. Plant so everything can be somewhat self—watered. Face plants south for full sun. Face southeast for partial shade, maximum warmth in the morning, and keeping cool in the afternoon heat.

Springs

Generally, find springs wherever you see a patch of coniferous trees or brush. You can either drink it straight from where it comes out, dig a whole to get to it, and/or make a man—made creek to direct it to the holding tank/cistern to use for cold drinking water, and to add to the volume of water coming down.

Either distill (boil, and separate steam from contaminates) drinking water, or use an ultra violet water purification filter to rid the water of any contaminants, and to minimize minerals, (as spring water is loaded with minerals, and can cause diarrhea).

FOODS

(**Note:**) The types of foods, herbs, plants, etc. listed here don't necessarily grow in every climate or environment, but generally for nutritional or medicinal purposes, there are substitutes.

- Fruits and Berries contain germicides, such as malic, tartaric, and citric acids, which disinfect and purify the system. Germs can't live or grow in fruit and berry juices. Once these acids are digested, they become highly alkaline in the body. Alkaline foods help prevent and treat illness, and flush the system of toxins.
- Oats have antiseptic properties, which also helps prevent and treat disease.
- Oats and nuts are high in carbohydrates, and unsaturated fats, which, along with honey, and fruit sugars, is the best source of energy there is. Though grains and starches take longer to digest, they also add to the time it takes before a refill of food energy is due.
- Nuts can easily replace meat and dairy products (except for vitamin B12 content); almonds and pecans have an alkaline reaction once ingested, and therefore they also help keep one's system pure.
- Eliminating meat (especially store—bought meat) and dairy products from the diet is the first thing that should be done if toxins and impurities are to be completely removed from the body. This aspect cannot be underestimated. Eating the flesh from dead animals has many negative effects on one's system, especially if one eats large quantities of meat and dairy products. Meat, dairy, and

animal products are high in cholesterol, and saturated fats, and may cause clogged arteries, poor circulation, constipation, high risk of heart failure/disease, strokes, varicose veins, hemorrhoids, high blood pressure, obesity, breast cancer, colon cancer, prostate cancer, pancreatic cancer, stomach cancer, cervical cancer, enodmetrial cancer, diabetes, hypoglycemia, peptic ulcers, hernias, diverticulosis, hypertension, asthma, salmonellosis, trichinosis, and the like. Meat contains numerous types of bacteria, parasites, and carcinogens, which can lead to cancer and infection. Meat always decays in a very short period of time. Eating too much meat can lead to rheumatism, kidney stones/diseases, gout, gallstones, and bright's disease. Women who eat a lot of meat increase their chances of developing breast cancer by ten times!

When the dead flesh of animals is ingested, there is generally too much protein in the body. When one consumes too much protein, it has to be stored somewhere, which ends up being in the blood. Excess protein becomes acidic, and the body will draw out calcium and magnesium from the bones and teeth to increase alkalinity in the blood to keep the Ph balance in check. So, in essence, excess protein (especially animal proteins) robs the bones and teeth of calcium and magnesium, which is the leading cause of osteoporosis. In fact, people (especially women) who eat meat and dairy products on a regular basis are actually doubling their chances of developing osteoporosis! Eating one steak cooked outside on a barbecue grill has the same cancer—causing effects as smoking 300 cigarettes! In the Christian bible, man could live up to one thousand years or more. When man introduced eating the flesh of animals into the diet, the lifespan had dramatically reduced…now down to less than one hundred years. Of course Christians blame the lifespan loss on man committing sins, but to look at it in a logical view, without considering religion…the timing is perfect. Before man started eating animals (living souls), he lived for about 1000 years. After man started eating flesh, he slowly but surely lost the original lifespan.

Though eliminating meat and dairy products from the diet will rid your system of impurities, vegetarians must be sure they are getting enough Vitamin B12 in the diet. Comfrey, (combined with dandelion, so there are no adverse side affects on the liver), V10 juice, barely gress, grains eaten with veggies, and the following foods will keep you healthy, and your nutrition up to snuff.

Nuts & Fruit: (dwarfing trees) almonds, apples, apricots, bananas, black cherries, brazil nuts, figs, peaches, pears, rose hips (see "Herbs" chapter), and cherry tomatoes (look below).

Growing Advice: Plant rootstocks in a sunny location, with some, but minimal shade. Water regularly. (As a general rule, plant more than one variety of each tree, for better crops, and cross—pollination). By using the dwarfing varieties, the trees should produce fruit by their second or third year. Not much pruning is needed, but the lowest branch should be about 6—12" above ground. Cut off sprouts, suckers, and broken ends. (Against a wall or trellis, the dwarf fruit tree can provide food and a simpler way of getting to it; not to mention, providing a sense of seclusion, to go along with a water garden, herb garden, and what have you.) Another recommendation is to pick off the small fruits every 6" or more, in order to provide a better crop the following year. Mulch with straw, or other organic material deep enough to smother grass and weeds. Keep a few inches away from the trunks to avoid mice. Apply fine wire mesh around trunk bases. (Almonds can be grown like bushes by keeping them pruned).

Cherry tomatoes
Growing advice: pretty simple—just read the back of the seed package.

Grapes
Growing Advice: (vining plant—use a rock wall, or trellis…not necessary to connect to a trellis until they grow tall enough. A stake will do until then). Prune tops back to a single cane, so that only two buds are left. Plant root canes about one foot deep, so that the buds are just above the soil. Prune every year. Harvest when birds start pecking at the fruit.

Berries

Blackberries
Growing Advice: Plant 1/2" root cuttings vertically 1 to 3 ft apart in 3 to 4" of loose, moist, rich soil. Compost. Harvest leaves and roots any time. Harvest berries in mid to late summer. For ease of harvesting, train branches along supports, and prune continuously. Full sun or partial shade.

Blueberries
Growing Advice: Plant root cuttings (more than one variety) in very acidic, rich, moist, well—drained soil. Mulch with acidic compost, not pine needles. Space 5 ft apart, with rows 7 ft apart.

Elderberries
Growing Advice: Plant seeds, or root cuttings in rich, moist soil in partial shade. You can hollow stems for small blowguns. (Larger stalks of other plants can be used for bigger blowguns—dry first). Can be dried and used as an insect repellant.

Raspberries
Growing Advice: Plant 1/2" root cuttings in a few inches of loose, rich, well—drained soil. Compost. Harvest leaves any time. Mature berries

appear in the summer. For ease of harvesting, train branches along supports, and prune mercilessly. Full sun or partial shade.

Strawberries: tonic, antioxidant, etc. (Use in facial creams, lotion, teas, etc.)

Growing Advice: Plant root cuttings in light, rich loam with plenty of humus, on a southern slope for better drainage. Strawberry bed should be cultivated 2 yrs before planting. Cut out any damaged or diseased leaves or keep damp, cool, and out of sun until planted. Plant vertically, 12—18" apart. Cover with 6" mulch/compost. Keep ever bearing varieties moist all summer. Create a barrier (as berry patches seem to take over) by laying out stone paths about 2 ½ feet wide, between growing beds (also 2 ½ feet wide). Winter protection, like straw or pine needles about 4" deep (loosen and remove in spring; reuse for summer; mulch after dried out).

Grains

Corn (dry the corn for horses, or pop corn…burn the cobs for potash, in the making of soap).

Growing Advice: pretty simple—follow the instructions on the seed package.

Oats

Growing Advice: Plant seeds in clay, loam—early spring. Harvest in 90 to 110 days. Cut to ground, tie stems, and hang upside down to dry. Beat heads in a funnel—shaped, weaved basket (top half open, for the path of strikes). Roll a metal bar across the tops to push off the rest of the grains. Return stems to growing bed, burn, and till. You could probably plant two crops in one year, but you should have a spring bed, and a summer bed. The spring bed would be the first crop, and you could use the stems for composting the summer bed, (which should have more shade, in a cooler place, and with about 1/2 to 1/3 daylight.), or weaving baskets.

Barley

Growing Advice: Same as oats, except it needs a little more fertile, well—drained soil; and you could use the same bed twice a year, in a cool, moist place. Also, save the stems and leaves. Cut some before they produce barley grain. They can be juiced, or dried/powdered and added to Nutri—Milk, tea, etc. "Barley Grass" is bombarded with nutrients and plant proteins.

Seeds

Sunflower
Growing Advice: Plant 1 ft apart, ½ " deep, in rich, moist, deeply cultivated, light loam. Sunflowers are ready for harvest as soon as the birds start picking the outer rows of seed; this method can be used in a lot of different plants to determine harvest time, and protect your share of the crop. Cut heads about 1 ft down the stalk. Tie stalks together and hang upside down to dry—as you would for herbs. (You could probably use the stalks for making whistles, if you dry them out first).

Sweetener

Honey (bees)
Production Advice: Use May and June flowers, and some clover through the summer; fall wild flowers through September and October. (For specific plant varieties, attracting bees, see the end of this section.) Have large empty hives ready for transferring the bees from their previous homes. Use an extractor to throw out the honey by centrifugal force; you can use the combs for wax (candles). Try the Italian type of bees. If any group of bees loses its queen, you will have to either wait for them to raise one or you will need to buy another one as a replacement. Increase hives from two, to four, to six, and so on.

Start with two colonies and two hive bodies; when one is filled, add another to give more room for production. When one colony dies, brush the dead bees from the combs, and scrape the whole hive clean and give the honeycombs to another bee colony. As fall approaches, gather the honey (in the upper portions only) and remove gradually, down to the bottom 1/3 to 1/2 portion of hives. (The rest of the honey should be left for the bees). Keep hives out of wind, and give winter protection. Reduce entrances to keep out rodents and help keep warm; wrap hives in a thick wool blanket and cover them with tarred building paper.

Plants that attract bees: basil, catnip, chamomile, hyssop, rosemary, sage, lavender, clover, and alfalfa. (Others may be used for a different taste, but may not be as attractive to bees).

Vegetables: Sweet peas, carrots, celery, parsley…

Sweet peas (vine type)
Growing Advice: Plant seeds 1—2" apart and 3" deep in the late fall, just before the ground is expected to freeze. Mound the soil slightly over the plants. As soon as the ground freezes hard, mulch. (Remove in spring). Needs rich, well—drained, well—cultivated soil, with well—rotted manure. Compost. Keep cool. Keep seedpods cut.

(The other veggies are easy to grow; just follow the directions on your seed packages).

Soybeans

Growing Advice: Plant seeds after the last frost; much like you would plant and cultivate a corn crop. You can let the soybeans/pods mature until dry. Then, you can grind them up, or store as is in a glass jar in a cellar. Soybeans are high in protein, contain twice the calcium of cow's milk, and can be a perfect substitution for meat and dairy products.

Storage

Fruit: Sundry, or freeze—dry. Do not mix fruit as it is drying.

Berries: (and grapes) place in plastic containers, and store in the freezer. If you freeze—dry them, store in a cellar afterward.

Grains, Nuts, Seeds, Barley, and Honey: Use for making granola, milk, sweeteners and the like. To store before using in recipes, just cover and place in a solar oven for about fifteen minutes, or until very light golden colored. Then, store in glass jars in the cellar as is, or grind into powders first for later use.

Juice (for soap, or just to drink): pulverize the fruit, berries, or veggies until they are at the desired thickness, then strain. Though a more preferable way is to use a juice press or an electric juicer. Either way, once the food/s are juiced, refer to the following examples to preserve the juices.

To freeze, just pour the juice into plastic baggies and leave in the freezer. To can the juices, so you can store them in a cellar, pour the juice into glass canning jars, leaving about ¼ to ½ inch space on top. Then, place the jars in a hot water bath.

Berry juice: @ 190 degrees for ½ hour
Cherry juice: @ 185 degrees for ½ hour
Grape juice: @ 190 degrees for ½ hour
Apricot nectar/juice: @ boiling for 15—20 minutes
Tomato juice: @ simmering/boiling for 15—20 minutes
Peaches, pears, and other high acid foods: @ boiling for ½ hour
Strawberries: @ simmering for 10—15 minutes

Note: always store dried foods in glass jars, or pottery with heavy lids in a cool, dark place, like a cellar. (Lids should be heavy enough that rodents can't get in...they should not have air leaks that will allow insects to get in).
Notes

To know about how much you should eat to be at a healthy weight, multiply your body weight by ten. (For example, if you weigh 200 lbs., you should consume 2000 calories/day. But, if you want to lose or gain weight, for instance: I weigh 100 lbs., but I want to gain weight. 100 lbs x 10 =1000 cal./day to remain 100 lbs. It takes 3500 calories to make one pound of fat. So, if every day, I take in 500 calories more than I burn up as energy, by the end of the week, I would have gained one pound; The same is true for losing weight, only instead of increasing calories, you would decrease them, or burn more up as energy, with exercise).

- Eat protein foods with sweat peas, but separate from granola, fruit, and berries, because when you combine protein foods with calcium foods (like nuts, figs, raisins), more calcium is excreted from the body, meaning less calcium for the bones and teeth.
- Always store dried foods in glass jars, or heavy pottery to keep out rodents, light, and moisture.

Note, that when fruits/veggies are juiced, the nutritional value is concentrated up to 30%; when dried, nutritional value is concentrated up to 40%, and still only weighs about ¼ of the weight of fresh foods.

Just so you get an idea of the differences between this type of a diet, and that of the average American diet:

- There are about 84.5 milligrams of Vitamin C in 1 Cup of strawberries, as opposed to 69.7 milligrams of Vitamin C in one orange. (Which amounts to about 1 cup as well).
- There are about 332 mg of Calcium in 1 Cup of almonds, compared with between 230—300 milligrams of Calcium in 1 Cup of milk. (See Recipe chapter for powdered Nutri—Milk recipe; easier method of digestion/good for pouring on granola, a bowl of cereal, or just to drink).
- Barley grass contains chlorophyll and is very rich in the following nutrients: potassium, calcium, magnesium, iron, copper, folic acid, pantothenic acid, phosphorus, manganese, zinc, beta carotene,

Vitamins B1, B2, B6, C, and 80 mg Vitamin B12 per 100 grams; Contains 11 times the calcium in cow's milk, 7 times the Vitamin C in oranges, and almost 5 times the iron in spinach. It is useful in treating bronchitis, and poor blood circulation as well.

None of the foods mentioned contain any cholesterol, except for fish, elk, and deer (animal products). Contrary to the notion that cholesterol is a very bad, and unhealthy thing, it is required for the formation of sex and adrenal hormones, vitamin D, and bile (which digests fats). Cholesterol also plays an important role in helping to keep the skin soft, and keeping the brain and nervous system functioning properly. Though cholesterol may have beneficial effects on one's system, too much can cause serious damage to the body, such as blocking arteries, and causing heart attacks and/or strokes. As in any case, too much of a good thing…well, I think you get the idea.

NUTRITION

Energy

Vegan Food Pyramid

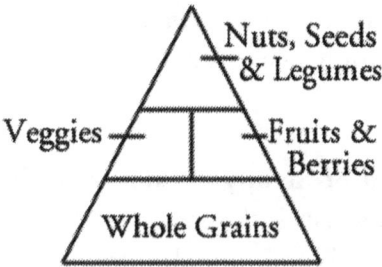

Carbohydrates are broken down into simple sugars, which are carried to the liver to be changed into glucose. This process makes it possible for glucose to be readily available to be used as energy. They help produce heat in the body, help break down fats, assist in digestion, is needed for fueling the brain tissues, nervous system, and muscles.

Types of sugars, and sources

Glucose—The only form of sugar that can be used by the body for producing energy. Present in fruits and honey.

Sucrose—The combination of glucose and fructose; the same as honey.

Fructose—Bypasses any other reduction processes of the body, and is automatically stored as fat; available in fruits, some vegetables, honey, and berries.

Maltose—Malt sugar, malting process of grains.

Starch—Changed into glucose. Takes longer to digest, but energy lasts longer, and it takes longer to feel hungry again. Available in grains, nuts, sunflower seeds, yams, and some veggies.

Fats give shape to various parts of the body, help regulate the body temperature, and provide a more concentrated form of energy, though the best sources of energy are obtained from carbohydrates. Fats are carriers of the fat—soluble vitamins, (such as Vitamins A, D, E, and K), and help the body absorb them.

Protein (comprised of mainly 22 amino acids) repairs, builds, and rebuilds body tissue. Protein is the main building blocks of forming hormones, hair, skin, nails, blood, muscles, and internal organs, (the heart and brain included). It is also a source of body heat, and energy.

- Too much protein in the diet inhibits calcium from being absorbed…so does laxatives and other medicines that cause diarrhea…as does excessive amounts of phosphorus.
- Parsley and some other foods contain calcium, but the body cannot absorb it because of the oxalic acid. Adding other foods containing calcium, and consumed at the same meal will work, though, because the oxalic acid inhibits the calcium in parsley, but doesn't affect other foods containing calcium.
- Combine Vitamin C foods with foods containing iron…Vitamin C increases absorption of iron and calcium, and converts the inactive form of folic acid into the active form.

■ Sprouting increases lysine, and triptophan, helps increase protein, Vitamins B, E, and K content, and Vitamin C is increased by as much as five times. To sprout alfalfa, oats, un—hulled sunflower seeds, barley, soybeans, or corn (among other grains): Place 1 tbs seeds in a quart—sized jar, and spray with water; cover the top of the jar with a clean nylon stocking, and secure with a rubber band. Pour off the water (good to use for houseplants), and rinse the seeds. Turn the jar on its side. Water the seeds two times daily, making sure to pour off remaining water, so they aren't continually soaking. Continue this process for about five or six days, giving them some, but minimal light. Refrigerate, or juice, and store.

■ Any excess in carbohydrates, fats, and/or protein is automatically stored as fat.

Recommended Daily Allowance

Nutrient	Amount needed	Best Sources
Carbohydrates	67 gm per 1000 calories	Oats, fruit (especially dried), veggies
Fats	33.5 gm per 1000 calories	Nuts, seeds
Protein	Body weight divided by 3	Oats, nuts, seeds, peas, alfalfa, some in fruits and veggies
Calories	Body weight x 10	
Vitamin A	4000-6000 IU	Carrots, tomatoes, cantaloupe, peaches, apricots, watermelon, alfalfa, comfrey, grapes, peaches, barley grass, dandelion, apples, berries, figs

Vitamin A	4000-6000 IU	Carrots, tomatoes, cantaloupe, peaches, apricots, watermelon, alfalfa, comfrey, grapes, peaches, barley grass, dandelion, apples, berries, figs
Vitamin B1	0.5 mg per 1000 calories	Oats, peas, nuts, seeds, alfalfa, comfrey, barley grass, soy beans
Vitamin B2	1.2 – 1.4 mg	Oats, nuts, alfalfa, comfrey, barley grass, soy beans
Vitamin B6	2 – 2.2 mg	Oats, nuts, seeds, alfalfa, comfrey, barley grass, soy beans
Vitamin B12	3 – 15 mcg	Comfrey, barley grass
Biotin	0.05 –0.30 mg	Oats, soybeans, elderberries, grapes, cantaloupe, peaches, raisins, raspberries, strawberries, watermelon, almonds, carrots
Niacin	13 NE	Oats, nuts, figs, bananas, comfrey, tomatoes
Pantothenic Acid	4 – 7 mg	Oats, comfrey, barley grass
Folic Acid	400 – 800 mcg	Oats, nuts, carrots, cantaloupe, barley grass
Vitamin C	35 – 100 mg	Tomatoes, strawberries, comfrey, cantaloupe, rosehips, dandelion, barley grass
Vitamin D	200 – 400 IU	Sunshine (10 to 15 min./day), alfalfa, comfrey
Vitamin E	12 – 15 IU	Oats, nuts, seeds, carrots, comfrey, soy beans
Calcium	800 – 1200 mg	Oats, nuts, figs, raisins, comfrey, barley grass, soy beans
Copper	2 – 3 mg	Oats, nuts, dried fruit, peas, barley grass
Iron	10 – 18 mg	Oats, nuts, raisins, dried fruit, barley grass, alfalfa
Magnesium	300 mg	Peas, apples, cherries, figs, raisins, alfalfa, celery, barley grass
Manganese	2.5 – 5 mg	Oats, nuts, barley grass
Phosphorus	800 – 1200 mg	Oats, nuts, comfrey, barley grass, alfalfa
Potassium	1825 – 5625 mg	Oats, dried fruit, bananas, comfrey, barley grass, alfalfa
Selenium	0.05 – 0.2 mg	Oats, nuts, barley grass
Sodium	1500 – 2500 mg	Strawberries, apples, cucumbers, alfalfa, carrots, celery, watermelon
Zinc	15 mg	Oats, nuts, barley grass
Cholesterol	Less than 300 mg	Animal products only, but if fatty foods (like nuts) are ingested, it helps the body make its own cholesterol

As you can see, plant foods, honey and herbs provide you with all of the energy, vitality, health, and the necessary daily nutritional requirements and thus, meat and dairy products can safely be eliminated from the diet. You could even live a very long and healthy life from only drinking the juices from these foods (with the inclusion of water as well).

Whether you choose to eat these foods fresh, freeze—dried, juiced, or in oat/nut milk preparations, even just one cup of oats, nuts, sunflower seeds, and a handful here and there of fresh and/or dried fruits, and veggies per day, will provide you with the daily caloric and nutritional requirements. The Nutri—Milk recipe is wonderfully balanced with soy, oat, nut, and sunflower seed milk. (Refer to the Recipes chapter). There are also many different juices you can prepare from fruits, berries, and veggies.

Raw and Uncooked

Raw, fresh, juiced, and uncooked living foods are the best source of nutrition there is. But, when winters are harsh, the next best thing would be foods that have been either juiced and canned, freeze—dried, or made into milk.

- **Freeze—dried** foods are first frozen, and then vacuum—dried. Since many nutrients (particularly Vitamins A, C, and E) are lost to heat, light, and oxidation, freezing the foods first, and sucking out the water content with vacuum pressure is the very best way to preserve these vitamins.
- **Reverse Osmosis** is basically like a water filter; only the holes from which the water passes through are much smaller. The water is forced through the filter, leaving the small, *dry* particles behind. This process can be used to make products such as powdered milk alternatives (like nut milks), powdered fruit/veggie juices, and such. The best thing about reverse osmosis is that it doesn't use heat, light, or hot air to obtain the powdered form of a liquid. This

way, nutrients are not lost to heat, light, or oxidation. Generally, you would add about 2 heaping tbs of powdered milk/juice to 8 oz water, more or less to suite your taste.

The best way to obtain the richest amount of nutrients, is to avoid/eliminate the following:

- ○ Cooking (# 1 nutrient murderer) or heating of any kind (especially above 120 degrees)
- ○ Exposure to sunlight
- ○ Exposure to air (use cotton balls to displace the air inside storage containers, when they aren't full)

You can store anywhere from four to eight times more freeze—dried/powdered foods, as opposed to whole or canned foods; and they will last for up to one year (more or less) compared to just a few days shelf/refrigerator life for whole or canned foods. Canned foods have a similar shelf life of freeze—dried foods as well, but as much as possible…fresh is best.

So to make it brief, fresh is best. But during the winter months and between growing seasons, freeze—dried/powdered foods, and those preserved by means of reverse osmosis are nearly equal in nutritional content as fresh foods. (About 95 to 99%).

Raw Foods Diet

A raw foods diet is most likely *the very best way* to sustain maximum health, and should not be underestimated. Drinking living food juices requires very little digestion, and is directly absorbed into the bloodstream. Drinking the juice or milk from plants not only prevents your system from being overtaxed, but also allows one to ingest quite a bit more of these life—giving properties, available in fresh, whole, living foods.

The idea here is that eating flesh from dead animals is simply not the way to "live long and prosper". In reality, the only way to beget *life*, is to eat living foods, with active nutrients. When you eat something dead, you can surely assume that all you will reap is what you've sewn.

Generally, when an animal is killed, it is hung until the blood stops running. The blood is the life of the animal. The meat is dead, and of course most people don't eat raw meat, as it can cause many illnesses. So meat eaters don't stop there, they have to cook the meat. When temperatures rise above 120 to 212 degrees, living nutrients are then dead, inactive, and cannot be used. So, when you sew the death of another animal, another living soul, then you will reap only deadly toxins and disease (which by consuming it, will eventually lead you to an early grave). If on the other hand, you sew the seeds of plants, to help them grow and live, you are contributing to their creation…their lives, and therefore your own. When you pick say an apple off a tree, or berries off a bush, it isn't killing them, nor harming them in any way. It's like getting a haircut, or cutting your nails, or shedding skin…harmless to the plant. Whether you pick the apple or not, the tree will continue producing them anyway. If you don't take the apple, it will be wasted, but hopefully the seeds will create new life. Think of it as a relationship similar to "the birds and the bees". When a flower produces pollen, bees will come take it to make food for a growing colony. In exchange for the pollen, the birds and the bees (among other animals) shake loose quite a bit of pollen as they fly, which will then fall to its destiny, and the pollen will eventually create a new generation of life from the original flower. In the same way, when we plant our orchards/gardens—to—be, we are not destroying life, but helping in the creation process. In exchange for the plants' lives being made possible, by our sewing of their seeds, they will give us healthy, life—giving foods to eat, positive energy, nutrition, and seeds in hope of yet another generation of their own kind.

In summary, living foods give life, while dead foods/flesh give death.

Note to meat eaters: I want you to know that I am not trying to attack your ways. If you think you need meat, by all means, do what you will with your own body. After all, this is a free country to some extent, correct? But, before you decide for sure that consuming animal products is right for you, maybe you should take a peeper at the following food facts.

Did You Know?

- Gelatin is made from boiled bones, skin, and tendons from animals
- Wine and canned bitter beer is made with isinglass (fish bladders), casein/potassium caseinate (milk proteins), and animal albumin (dried blood powder)
- Vodka is passed through bone charcoal
- With the average population of about 243,000,000 people in the United States, 60,000,000 of them die of starvation every year. 40,000 children starve to death every day, and all of these people could be saved if Americans would reduce their intake of meat and animal products by only 10%.
- Someone dies of a heart attack every 45 seconds, most of whom are meat eaters. In fact, anyone who eats meat on a consistent basis has a 50% chance of dying from a heart attack. Eating just one whole egg per day can increase your risk for heart attack by as much as 24%.
- Women who eat a meat based diet are subject to four times the risk of developing breast cancer than vegan women; and those of which who eat eggs, and butter/cheese obtained from dairy products have three times the risk of acquiring breast and ovarian cancer than vegan women.
- Men who eat a meat based diet are more than 3 and a half times more susceptible to prostate cancer than vegan men.
- 20% of caucasians and 80% of blacks have no lactase in their intestines, and are unable to digest dairy products anyway.

- Certain milk producer's original add campaign, "Everyone Needs Milk" was considered to be "False, misleading, and deceptive", according to the Federal Trade Commission.
- 94% of all animal products in the United States are contaminated with DDT, leaving meat—eating mothers with nearly 99% of the breast milk they feed their babies contaminated as well. Meat eating mothers have 35 times the amount of DDT in their milk as vegan mothers.
- The average sperm count for college students has declined by about 30%, due to DDT levels in their systems. The Meat Board tells us not to worry about the DDT, dioxins, and other pesticides contaminating our animal products, because they say "the quantities are so small"…and yet, a single ounce of it can kill 10,000,000 people.
- 20% of the cows in America are infected with the leukemia virus, and the highest rates of leukemia in children are found in the children who consume the most dairy products.
- Less than 1 in 250,000 animals are tested for toxic chemicals, with at least 500,000 animals being slaughtered for meat every hour.
- Out of the 125 medical schools in the United States, only about 30 of them require courses in nutrition; the average doctor only spends about 2 ½ hours of their time learning about nutrition.
- 55% of our livestock are routinely fed antibiotics, which is causing the effectiveness of antibiotics to decline rapidly…91% of the staphylococci infections in 1988 were resistant to antibiotics.
- The UK had to ban imported meat/animal products, and the use of feeding dead cows to each other, because of illnesses such as Mad Cow's Disease; and even though we have seen the devastation caused by this, America still supports the act of using dead animals to feed the living ones. The only difference here, is that we have banned feeding dead cows to live cows, but have allowed the act of feeding dead pigs and such to dead cows, and vise versa. Now, we

are finding out that new strains of Mad Cow's Disease are on the verge of becoming an epidemic in the U.S., including a new strain of a similar disease infecting our elk and deer. Why can't we learn from their mistakes, instead of blaming each other and pointing the finger? Who cares where it started, or who started it? What should be more important, is putting an end to the diseases once and for all.

- Europe has also banned the use of feeding antibiotics to their livestock, though the American meat and pharmaceutical industries give full and complete support. Obviously, there must be good reasons for Europe banning the use of feeding antibiotics to their livestock as well.

- With so many animals being grown/used for human consumption, we are polluting the air we breathe (30,000,000 tons of methane gas contributing to global warming), more of our water, the earth we stand upon, and the energy we need (10 times more energy used to produce/transport livestock, compared with veggies). We are essentially throwing our resources away, and killing our planet, all so we can eat the flesh of dead animals. What a waste!

- It takes five pounds of plant proteins to produce only one pound of protein from chicken flesh; it takes seven and a half pounds of plant proteins to produce only one pound of protein from hog flesh.

- 20 vegans could be fed on the amount of land it would take to feed 1 meat eating person.

- One acre of U.S. trees are lost every eight seconds to create crop land for livestock; just one person who switches to a vegan diet can save one acre of trees every year.

- Livestock consumes more than half of all the water used by the United States. It only takes 25 gallons of water to produce 1 pound of wheat, whereas it takes 2500 gallons of our water to produce 1 pound of meat…and we wander where our water supply is going to come from if we have a drought.

- The cost of hamburger meat would be $35/lb, if the water used by livestock weren't being paid for with American tax dollars. The average beefsteak would cost us $89/lb, if we weren't paying for the water used by livestock with our tax dollars.
- 1,000,000,000 tons of un—recycled waste is produced each year by livestock, much of which is dumped into our water supplies, filtered, and reused.
- If all Americans ate a meat centered diet, our petroleum reserves would only last for about 13 years, whereas if we were all vegans, our petroleum reserves would last for about 260 years. (Shipping, trucking, etc.).

How can switching to a vegan diet make any difference in how many lives are saved each and every year, due to disease and starvation? Well for starters, 1,300,000,000 people could be fed by the amount of grain and soybeans fed to the livestock.

So, before you feast your eyes on a big chunk of dead flesh, maybe you should consider all of the lives, including your own, that you could save by switching to a vegan diet. The next time you wander where our resources are going, maybe you should take a look at your plates. (No offense).

You Are What You Eat

Food gives us energy to grow. It may take some time getting used to the foods listed here, but if you grow your own food and consume only natural foods, eventually, you will come to appreciate yourself for growing your own food, and the food itself will prove to be more valuable to you. Not only will you develop a taste for these foods, but you will also be able to maintain a healthy and desirable weight, your brain will have sufficient fuel to function to the best of its ability, your mind will function better, your immune system and over all health will be enhanced, you will have more energy, more muscle; and your susceptibility to disease, illness, and physical stress will be greatly reduced. *Trust me…your body will thank you for it.*

RECIPES

Soap recipes: (2—6 oz medicinal herb, and 2—6 oz aromatic plant)

- Add catnip, hops, chamomile, yarrow, motherwort, and/or passionflower to calm, help induce sleep, relieve stress, or use marijuana oil (butter) for one of the oil bases.
- Add anise, feverfew, white willow, and/or red clover to help relieve menstrual pain.
- Add mint, basil, dill, hyssop, lavender, rosemary, and/or sage, to revive.

(**Note:** for visual purposes, you can extract the oil first, and add remnants to the soap along with the oil later).

Note: most of the specific amounts of each oil, herb, etc., will come from experiments, and should be written down as you learn (for aromatic purposes, you should try to experiment on which flowers/herbs to use as well). For reference as to which flowers/herbs to use, see Herb chapter. For a general idea, you would combine an average ratio of 12—16 oz potash, (with soaps and cleansers), 32 oz water, 48 oz almond oil, 38 oz brazil nut oil, and 2 to 6 oz aromatic plant oil. (If measured/poured into about 5 oz—volume soap molds, you would end up with about 27 bars of soap...enough to last a family of four for one year, more or less).

Toothpaste

Instructions: dehydrate, and grind the following ingredients into a fine powder; combine. To use, just add enough water to make a paste.

- 3 oz Bone meal (ground bones)—phosphorus, calcium, and fluoride
- 1 oz Dill seed—prevents bad breath; antiseptic properties
- 3 oz Mints—prevents tooth decay and kills bacteria
- 3 oz Myrrh—antiseptic, cures bad breath, helps fight bacteria that cause tooth decay; helps with bleeding gums, mouth ulcers, and sore throats (use in mouth washes too).
- 2 oz Hops—bacterial antibiotic
- 1 oz Alfalfa—source of chlorophyll; prevents bad breath
- 2 oz Comfrey—calcium, phosphorus, prevents cold sores

Aromatic and medicinal tea recipes

- To induce sleep, relieve stress, calm, etc: catnip, hops, chamomile, motherwort, marijuana, passionflower, and yarrow.
- To reduce menstrual pain: anise, red clover, and feverfew.
- To revive: mints, basil, dill, hyssop, lavender, rosemary, and sage.
- For PMS: juniper berry.
- To treat urinary tract infection: dill.
- To treat colds, coughs, flu, sore throat, headaches, and congestion: pennyroyal, rose, sage, meadowsweet, echinacea, mints, mullein, feverfew, anise, basil, rosemary, and pine needles.
- For a Tonic (To boost the immune system): red clover blossoms, chamomile, hops, hyssop, lavender, meadowsweet, raspberry leaves, sage, yarrow, comfrey, dandelion, alfalfa, and rosehips.
- To help prevent disease: juniper.

For additives (aroma/flavor purposes): add honey, and/or flowers (see herb section).

Note: For aromatic purposes, and external use: extract the oils. For herbal, and internal use: just dry, and use as necessary.

- Dry, and grind into a fine powder for lip balms, salves, paints, dyes, etc.
- Dry and crush for teas.

Basic Salve

Combine 4 oz dried herb to 1.5 lbs almond oil, and 4 oz beeswax, cover, and solar bake for three or four hours. Store in a dark, cool place, like a cellar. Once cooled, it will be firm and ready for use.

Menthol rub

Instructions: make a salve with plenty of mint oils added. No need for other herbs/flowers, but you can if you want.

Ingredients: 2 tbsp mint oil, 3 cups nut oil, and ½ cup beeswax.

Lip balm

Ingredients: 2 cups dried herb, 3 cups nut oil, and 1/2 cup beeswax...add hyssop, mint, and echinacea. You can add others if desired, but these would be the main ingredients.

Malt syrup

Instructions: extract the oil/butter from dried/powdered barley like you would for herbs/flowers, marijuana, etc. Take the clear fluid on top, and boil it down to the consistency of syrup.

Note: Barley malt is basically just barley sprouts.

Granola

Dry, grind, and combine two parts oats, 1 part nuts, equal parts (½ cup, per cup nuts) sunflower seeds and soy flour. Roll oats and flour in honey, malt honey, some chopped nuts, nut butter, nut oil, and whole sunflower seeds. Oven bake @ 400 degrees, or solar bake until golden brown; stir occasionally. Let cool, and store in cellar (in heavy pottery or plastic bags). After cooling, you can add carob chips, raisins, or any other dried fruit along with the granola mixture.

Lotion Recipe

The following recipe is meant to help the following:

- Moisturize, soothe, and tighten the skin
- Prevent/treat eczema (dry, scaly skin)
- Prevent/treat arthritis (stiff, sore joints)
- Promote good blood circulation (cold hands, feet, etc.)
- Prevent/treat acne
- Repel insects
- Promote melanin production and secretion (which protects your skin from ultraviolet light, and helps quicken the sun tanning process, safely)

Ingredients

38 oz pecan oil, 30 oz water, 40 oz almond oil, 8 oz sunflower seed oil, and 4 oz bee's wax, combined with the following:

Feverfew, oat milk, almond milk, basil, parsley, carrot juice, meadowsweet, aloe vera, chamomile, comfrey, dandelion, elder flowers, pennyroyal oil, rose oil, raspberry leaves/berries, strawberry leaves/berries, yarrow, and anise seed oil.

- Have all ingredients ready for use. Heat up beeswax, water, and nut oils to equal temperatures, so that everything is melted, and in liquid form.
- Add carrot juice, aloe vera gel, rose oil, anise seed oil, sunflower seed oil, oat milk, almond milk, pennyroyal oil, and any other liquid, aromatic ingredients you decide to add. (Keep all ingredients hot enough to stay liquid.)
- Add remaining ingredients (dried, and finely ground)
- Mix well, until all seems as one liquid. If there are any pieces of herb, or other ingredient, strain. (You would have to push the mixture through a strainer or coffee filter, because it should be somewhat thick).
- Pour mixture into containers, let cool, and store in cellar.

Note: If mixture is or isn't thick enough, add or don't add water…in step one, only add about half the amount given in the recipe. After you finish step 4, add as much water as necessary, to achieve desired thickness. (Remember, it will thicken more as it cools).

- Antioxidants, such as Vitamins A, C, and E help preserve the life of new skin cells, thereby slowing the effects of aging, such as dry, thin, or wrinkled skin.
- Tyrosine is synthesized from phenylalanine, which the body produces from the foods we eat, and is the pre—curser to melanin production.

- Melanin is the main amino acid responsible for protecting your skin from the harmful effects of ultra violet light; in the process of melanin production and secretion, the pigment of your skin darkens, resulting in what we call...a suntan. In other words, this lotion will also help you get a good tan, without burning your skin.
- Including sunflower seed oil with lotions, soaps, and skin products, provides a source of Vitamins A, D, and E...good for skin and preventing wrinkles.

Berry Tonic Tea

Ingredients: blackberries, strawberries, echinacea, hyssop, mints, juniper berry, rosehips, sage, raspberry leaves, and lavender. Juice the berries. Use dried herb, etc. held together with a piece of cloth, with a tie around the top. Steep in boiling berry juice instead of water.

- **To help prevent illness:** If anyone in your household (or anyone that you cannot avoid) gets sick, drink 4 cups of Juniper berry juice/tea per day. One before each meal, and one right before going to bed, until they aren't sick any more; or, use at the first sign of getting sick.

Note: only use juniper berry in tonic tea to prevent illness...not as a part of the everyday diet.

Malt Honey

Instructions: boil one pound finely ground oats (oat flour) in eight quarts of water, until mixture is thick. Once the starch is cooked, cool to between 140 and 170 degrees. Add two oz powdered barley malt, or malt syrup. (Barley malt is the sprouts, like alfalfa sprouts). Stir. Let stand until it tastes sweet. When the water is clear, strain out the thick mixture, and boil the liquid down to the consistency of syrup.

Apple Cider

Instructions: Juice your apples, and pour into clean glass jars or jugs, and stuff the openings with cotton wool plugs. (Don't stuff too tight). Let stand at room temperature for about 10 days, clean off the openings, and replace the cloths with wooden corks.

Note: This is the dry, alcoholic version, but it doesn't hurt to drink a little now and again, even for kids. (Not that you should go get your kid/s drunk, but it's actually quite healthy to drink about a cup or so a day).

To prevent fermentation, (non-alcoholic version), set in 165 degree hot water bath (simmering) for ½ hour, before allowing to sit at room temperature. You may want to strain the juice before serving.

Apple Cider Vinegar

Instructions: Pour apple cider into dark colored jars, leaving ¼ inch space on top. Cover with light woven cloth, such as a clean sheet, etc. Secure the top with a rubber band, and store in cellar for 4—6 months. Taste after four months; if it isn't ready, wait a month or two and test it again, until it is at the desired strength. Strain; pour in bottles/jars, and seal. Save the scum you strained out, so you can use it to strengthen your next batch by adding it to the mixture before allowing it to set in the cellar.

Fruit Leather

Instructions: After juicing your fruit and berries, you can use the pulp to make fruit leather. To do this, simply plop the pulp on a sheet of wax paper, place another sheet of wax paper on top of that, and flatten it out with a rolling pin. Roll it out as thin or as thick as you want. Take off the top layers of wax paper, and set in the sun until it is completely dehydrated.

Soy Milk

Ingredients:
2 cups soybeans
6 cups boiling water

Instructions: Soak soybeans overnight (8—12 hrs). Pour out water and rinse. Blend beans in 4 cups of boiling water. Strain the mixture through clean/thin sheet material. To make sure there will be no gritty mash particles in the finished product, you may want to try straining through one layer of sheet material, then two, and so on. Pour remaining two cups of boiling water through the pulp, allowing the milk to drip through your material, and into a cast iron skillet. Once all has dripped into the skillet, close the sheet material at the top, and squeeze out as much milk from the pulp as you can.

Bring milk to a boil. As the mixture begins to boil, stir occasionally with a spatula to prevent sticking on the bottom of the skillet. Boil over medium high heat for 1/2 to 1 hour. The longer it is boiled, the thicker and richer the milk will be.

Once finished with the above process, pour the milk into a jug, or jar, and refrigerate. Finally, add the following ingredients:

- 1 tbs vanilla extract, (vanilla is said to revive the brain and mind, increase muscular energy, and is considered an aphrodisiac)
- 2 tbs honey
- 2 tbs malt honey

- ¼ cup carob flour (optional)
- 1 tsp sunflower seed oil (cold pressed)
- 1 tsp almond oil (cold pressed)
- Blend well before storing in jugs or jars.
- Makes about 1 Quart.

Vanilla/Carob Malt Nutri Milk

Follow the Soy Milk recipe above to make soymilk; use the same recipe to make almond, oat, brazil nut, and sunflower seed milks. Make equal amounts of each, but make them separate. For the oat milk, you may only need to boil it for just 5 to 15 minutes. (Oat milk will thicken easily). For the sunflower seed, almond, and brazil nut milks, there is no need to cook after blending…just strain through clean, thin sheet material, pour in their containers, and chill. The time it takes to boil the oat milk depends on whether or not you roll the oats first. Grain mills, and rollers are not hard to obtain, and are very efficient for this process. Personally, I prefer the old fashioned manual stone mills, that you connect to your counter top, over the electric type, but either one will do fine. Nuts are better in nutritional quality when used immediately after the shelling process; to do this more efficiently, you should consider purchasing an electric nut sheller…nuts can be shelled in a much smaller amount of time, without the hassle and sore hands.

Once your nuts are shelled, your seeds are hulled, your oats are rolled, and your milks are made, combine the following ingredients:
- 1 Quart (4 Cups/Half Gallon) Soy Milk
- 1 Quart Oat Milk
- 1 Quart Sunflower Seed Milk
- 2 Cups (1 Pint/Half Quart) Almond Milk
- 2 Cups Brazil Nut Milk
- 3 Tbs Freeze-dried/powdered Barley Grass

- 1 Cups Carob Powder/Flour (optional—for a chocolate taste…additional calcium)
- Fruit Punch and/or cherry juice (optional—for a cherry/berry /fruity taste…additional nutrients)

Combine equal parts of the ingredients above together in a blender, 2 Cups at a time, and blend on high for a couple of minutes. Pour out the mixture, into a temporary large bowl. Repeat this process for the rest of the milk. You may want to strain the milk again, through some clean, thin sheet material for a smoother texture. Now, pour the milk into a jug or jar, and chill well before serving. You can either store the container of milk in a refrigerator, or in a very cool stream in the shade. Just be sure the container is sealed, airtight, watertight, and that it isn't exposed to sunlight. (Antioxidants are destroyed by heat, light, and oxygen).

Note: Can add a banana to the oat milk before combining with the rest of the ingredients, for a richer taste, and a thicker, smoother texture. Although, if you do add the banana, your milk will spoil quicker than if you don't add it…alternatively, you can add more oil, and/or cook the oat milk longer. To thin your milk, just add some water to the finished milk, (should be in a covered/sealed container), and shake well. To add more malt flavor, add malt honey; to add a carob/chocolate flavor, add carob powder; to add more vanilla flavor…experiment until you get the perfect blend of flavors, and the perfect taste and texture to suit your fancy (and your family's overall preference).

Note: Can choose from vanilla, carob malt, fruit, and cherry/berry flavors.

Makes about 1 ¼ Gallons, give or take, depending on whether you choose to include the carob flour, fruit punch, etc. or not.

Note: Do not blanch the nuts, or worry too much about oat husks, as you will lose some of the nutritional content by excluding them from the milk making process, especially the B vitamins. (Don't worry, you're going to strain the nut skins and oat husks out anyway).

Serving size: 1 ½ Cups

This drink accounts for over and above 2000 calories, because so many are used up and burned during the day with exercise. You burn up calories by consuming energy even at night when you are asleep, because the brain, nervous system, heart and such, need the calories to continue functioning at all…even if you aren't moving any part of your body, the involuntary muscles in the body need the extra energy. If you are a person with a slow metabolism and seem to gain weight even by the looks of food, you may only need just a few glasses a day. And, of course, if you are a child or teenager, you should only take in from 3 to 4 servings per day.

Vanilla Rice Pudding

1 Cup cooked brown rice
1 Cup nut, seed, or soy cream
2 to 3 Cups Nutri—Milk
½ to 1 Cup malt honey
1 ½ Tbs oat flour

½ to 1 tsp nutmeg
½ tsp cinnamon
¼ Cup carob powder (optional)
1 Tsp vanilla flavoring

Combine the cooked rice with carob flour (if you want chocolate pudding), stirring until melted. Beat the cream, malt honey, nutri—milk, oat flour, nutmeg, cinnamon, and vanilla in a bowl until smooth. Gradually beat this mixture into the rice. Stir/cook continuously over medium heat for 5 to 7 minutes. (Do not boil). Cover and chill.

Note: Can mix in some raisins, and/or chopped nuts after the pudding has cooled off.

For a chocolate flavored pudding, add the carob powder, use carob flavored Nutri—Milk instead of the vanilla flavored milk, and omit the cinnamon.

Fruit Salad

2 stalks sliced Celery (optional)   1 Apple cut in small pieces
½ Cup Grapes (cut in half)   ½ Cup chopped nuts
2 sliced Bananas   handful of sunflower seeds
½ Cup berries (your choice)   6 oz yogurt

Mix all ingredients, chill and serve.

Nut/Soy Butter

1 Cup water   1 ½ Cup nut oil
2 tbs powdered soybeans   ½ Cup sunflower seed oil

Mix and bring soy powder and water to a boil in a cast iron skillet. Strain, and pour ingredients in a bowl, including the oil. Beat constantly until thick, and store in a refrigerator.

Non Dairy Yogurt (after the first batch)

1 1/3 Cups powdered Nutri—Milk   2 Cups water

Instructions: Heat evenly over medium heat, stirring often until hot, but not boiling. Let cool for an hour; add 2 large tbs store—bought plain yogurt, and mix well. Cover and set in the sun for 8 hrs. Refrigerate/chill and serve plain, add fruit and/or berries, or use in a Fruit Smoothie. Save a couple of tbs of the yogurt for the next batch.

Nut Butter Granola Bars

- 1 ½ Cups Carob Chips
- 1 Cup Peanut, Almond, and/or Brazil Nut Butter
- ½ Cup Soy Butter
- 1 Cup Chopped Nuts
- 2 Cups Oats
- 1 Cup Sunflower Seeds
- 1 Cup Honey

Instructions: Place the Soy Butter and Nut Butters in a bowl, and heat on high in a microwave until melted. Add oats, nuts, seeds, and honey. Squish into a baking dish and just chill baby. (Refrigerate). Before the mixture sets completely, squish the carob chips into the top. Let the mixture continue to chill until set. Finally, cut the granola into bars, and serve. (Store any left ovaries in the cellar…maybe even the right ones too).

Fruit Museli

- 1/3 Cup Oats
- ½ Cup Vanilla Nutri—Milk
- Some Chopped Nuts
- ¼ Cup Raisins
- Several Grapes
- 1 Apple
- Some dried fruit cut into small pieces (your choice)

Instructions: Combine oats, nuts, milk, and raisins in a covered container, and refrigerate over night. In the morning, grate the apple, cut the dried fruit, slice the grapes in half, and add to the mixture. Stir well, and serve.

Makes about 1 serving.

Fruit Smoothie

- 1 Cup Fresh Fruit (bananas, peaches, cantaloupe, and possibly pears)
- 1 Cup Frozen Fruit (Grapes/Berries-strawberries, blackberries, blueberries, raspberries, elderberries, etc).
- ½ Cup Vanilla Nutri—Milk
- ½ Cup Apple Juice or Fruit Punch

Combine all the ingredients together, and blend on high until at desired texture. You can also add a touch of honey, or barley malt honey/syrup.

Fruit Punch

- ¼ Cup of each of the following ingredients:

apple juice, grape juice, blackberry juice, blueberry juice, raspberry juice, strawberry juice, cantaloupe juice, and pear juice.

Combine the ingredients, add some ice cubes, and blend thoroughly. Chill, and serve.

Makes about 1 ¾ Cups per serving.

Here is an *example* of a **Healthy Diet Plan:**

Breakfast: 2 Servings Vanilla Nutri—Milk poured over granola, with a small glass of peach nectar. Can add dried fruit, such as raisins, chopped/dried apples, etc. in the granola cereal.

Or—Fruit Museli, with 2 Servings Vanilla Nutri—Milk poured over top, and a small glass of peach nectar.

Brunch: Nut Butter Granola Bars and 1 Serving Carob, or Fruit flavored Nutri—Milk

Or—2 ½ Cups fruit punch, a couple of handfuls of dried fruits, and 1 serving Nutri—Milk (your choice of flavor)

Or—1 serving fruit punch flavored Nutri—Milk, and a couple of handfuls of dried fruits

Lunch: A few handfuls of dried fruits, 1 serving fruit punch flavored Nutri—Milk, and a handful or two of cherry tomatoes

Or—Fruit Salad, 1 serving Fruit Punch, several dried figs, and a handful or two of cherry tomatoes

Or—Fruit Smoothie/Fruit flavored Nutri—Milk, several dried figs, and a handful or two of cherry tomatoes

Linner/Afternoon: Nut Butter Granola Bar and 1 Serving Carob Malt Nutri—Milk, or Fruit/Berry/Cherry flavored Nutri—Milk

Or—1 serving hot carob milk, and some fruit leather, or dried fruit

Dinner: A handful of fresh veggies (optional), 3 Cups Carrot/Veggie Juice

After Dinner: 1 serving Vanilla, Carob Malt, or Fruit/Berry/Cherry flavored Nutri—Milk, or hot carob (like hot chocolate, only just heat up some carob flavored Nutri—Milk, pour in a mug, and sprinkle marsh mallows on top).

- If you are an adult, on a 2000 calorie diet or more, try to drink about five servings Nutri—Milk daily.
- Drink 1 to 3 cups mint tea daily, to prevent gas/diarrhea (if you are just started on this diet, and are used to being constipated/eating meat…especially if you quit cold turkey. Although, I quit eating animal products cold turkey, and had no trouble with gas or diarrhea…just a precaution).
- Always be sure to brush your teeth as soon as possible after eating dried fruits, because they stick to your teeth, and have high levels of fruit sugar

I would have to say, the two best reasons for sticking to a diet of this sort, would be:

1-This diet alone provides over and above 2000 calories, all complete proteins and amino acids, carbohydrates, fats, minerals, vitamins, and all nutritional requirements necessary to sustain maximum bodily health and energy in every way. Some people have trouble losing weight, or keeping it off, and should therefore be sure to exercise plenty to burn off those extra calories, and possibly limit their servings to 4 per day. Other people, (like me), have trouble gaining weight, or keeping it on, and should possibly consider drinking one more serving of Nutri—Milk daily. Generally, 4 to 6 servings should be sufficient.

2-As long as you store all foods immediately after harvest, you would hardly every have to cook!! All you would have to do in this respect is to make up a batch of Nutri—Milk every other morning, and make your fruit museli the night before you want it. Everything else would be supplied either fresh, frozen, powdered, or freeze-dried. Eating healthy is as simple as you make it. All the hassle people and restaurants go through, to cook their foods isn't even worth the trouble. All it does is deplete the food of its nutrients, and kill any living proteins/amino acids, making them un-usable to the body.

Note: It may take some time for your body to get used to this type of a diet; when you are used to lots of meats, cheeses, eggs, and dairy products, you are also probably used to only about 1 bowel movement in a matter of about 2 days. When you begin eating foods which contain natural fibers, more than likely for the first couple or few weeks, you will have more like 2 or 3 bowel movements per day. I know, this may sound gross, but what goes in must come out...and wouldn't you rather that it comes out with-out any hassles, or need for newspapers in the bathroom, or enemas?

Also be sure to drink at least 2 to 3 Cups of water daily (since you will be getting about 3 ¼ Cups water in 5 servings of Nutri—Milk, and 1 to 4 Cups water in the tea per day...as long as the water adds up to about 8 cups). This will keep your energy levels up, and will prevent dehydration.

If you would like to try this kind of milk without the hassle of making it yourself, look for Pacific Foods Products. They supply us with nutri-tional drinks like multi-grain milk, original or vanilla oat milk, enriched cocoa, coffee, plain, or strawberry soy milk, original, cocoa, plain, or vanilla flavored rice milk, original or vanilla flavored almond milk, vanilla or cocoa flavored naturally complete (combined) milks, organic carrot juice, bone health mixed berry smoothies, and many more different types of natural beverages. The company also has a website at *www.pacific-foods.com*. I have to say, their products, along with Silk Milk products are the very best tasting alternative milks I have tried...and I have tried many.

HERBS

Alfalfa: arthritis, helps neutralize and rid the body of carcinogens, bad breath, asthma, hay fever, promote menstruation, vitamins A, E, K, B, and D; high in protein, contains phosphorus, iron, magnesium, chlorine, sodium, silicon, potassium; helps digestion, gas, ulcers, dropsy, obesity, mild laxative, tonic, stomachic, diuretic.

Growing Advice: Plant seeds in deep loam, water well, and use manure to help feed it. If you have a large field of alfalfa, use a tractor to cut it when the plants are green and mature. Use the remains for composting…high in nitrogen. (Parts used—roots and leaves)

Aloe: antiseptic, burns, fungal antibiotic, poison ivy, dry skin, and chapped lips.

Growing Advice: Three parts sandy loam, one part gravel. Compost. Water very little, except when growing rapidly. Low humidity, plenty of sun, can't handle temperatures below 40 degrees. (Parts used—gel)

Anise: stimulant, tonic, asthma, cough, decongestant, gas, menopausal discomforts, menstrual discomforts, nausea. (Parts used—seeds and roots)

Growing Advice: Plant seeds 1/8" deep in rich, well—drained soil, with full sun. Germination takes about 1 or 2 weeks @ about 70 degrees. 18" apart. Shelter from wind. Harvest when seeds are green to grayish brown, cutting entire flower head before seed clusters break open. Collect flowers in a bag to prevent seed scatter.

Apple: antiseptic, bacterial antibiotic, constipation, diarrhea, food—poisoning treatment, laxative. (Parts used—fruit)

Growing Advice: (see Food>Nuts & Fruit section…dwarfing trees)

Basil: stimulant, aromatic, immune system stimulant, insect bites/stings, parasitic antibiotic, snakebites, stomach cramps, vomiting. (Parts used—leaves, flower tops)

Growing Advice: Plant seeds 1/8" deep in well—drained soil, full sun. Compost. 1 ft apart. Mulch. Prune every few weeks.

Blackberry: antiseptic, bleeding, tonic, diarrhea, hemorrhoids, mouth sores, wounds. (Parts used—leaves, bark, roots, fruit)

Growing Advice: (see Food>Berries section).

Catnip: antiseptic, anxiety, bacterial antibiotic, food—poisoning treatment, stress, tranquilizer. (Parts used—flowers, leaves)

Growing Advice: Plant seeds in well—drained soil. Full/mostly sun. 18" apart. Harvest when in bloom.

Chamomile: antiseptic, antiviral, anxiety, arthritis, bacterial antibiotic, bladder trouble, bronchitis, burns, expel worms, food—poisoning treatment, fungal antibiotic, immune system stimulant, increases appetite, jaundice, kidneys, prevent gangrene, regulate periods, stress, tonic, colds, bronchitis, aromatic, tranquilizer, ulcer prevention/treatment, wash for open sore/wounds, yeast infections. (Parts used—flowers)

Growing Advice: Scatter seeds on well—prepared beds, in sandy, well—drained soil. Gently tap down. Partial shade. Flowers for several weeks. Harvest when in bloom.

Comfrey: one of the very few plant sources known containing Vitamin K, and B12…also contains good amounts of Vitamins B1, B2, B6, D, and E; leaves are rich in Vitamins A, and C, among other nutrients; wound healing, digestive aid, emollient, astringent, coughs, kidneys, stomach, bowels, bloody urine, eczema, anemia, gall and liver diseases, hemorrhoids, strengthens blood, cleanses entire system of impurities, bruises, sores, boils, bleeding gums. (Parts used—roots and leaves).

Growing Advice: Plant inch—long root cuttings 3" deep, in well—drained soil. Allow full sun, or partial shade. Plant 3 ft apart. Border with stone paths (1 ft deep). Leaves may be harvested when flowers begin to bud. Gather roots in the autumn, after the first frost, or in spring before the first leaves appear. Wash roots thoroughly and cut in slices to dry. Powder, and store in sealed container.

Dandelion: kidney and liver disorders, skin diseases, fevers, hepatitis, gout, stiff joints, contains insulin substitutes needed by diabetics, snake bites, warts, high vitamin/mineral content, pms, high blood pressure, cancer prevention, vitamins A and C, yeast infection, possible arthritis treatment…Be sure to eat foods with plenty of potassium (long term use depletes this nutrient.) (Parts used—mostly roots, but also leaves)

Growing advice: No need to explain…they grow everywhere. Most people consider them annoying, pesky weeds.

Dill: aromatic, stimulant, bacterial antibiotic, diarrhea, gas, food—poisoning treatment, urinary tract infection treatment. (Parts used—seeds)

Growing Advice: Plant seeds ¼" deep, in rich, moist, slightly acidic soil. Place 12" apart, in a sunny location. (Fresh dill is much more aromatic.) Seeds mature in about two months. Harvest when they begin to turn brown. Self—sows. (Leave a few plants un—harvested).

Echinacea: bacterial antibiotic, fungal antibiotic, antiseptic, protozoan antibiotic, anti—inflammatory, immune system stimulant (tonic), arthritis, bronchitis, burns, colds and flu, cold sores, ear infection, food—poisoning treatment, psoriasis, whooping cough, wounds, yeast infections, blood poisoning, fevers, acne, insect stings, snake bites, gangrene, tonsillitis, sores. (Parts used—roots)

Growing Advice: Tamp seeds into moist, slightly acidic, sandy soil when weather is in the 70's. Full sun. It takes four years for roots to grow large enough to harvest. Pull them in autumn after plant has gone to seed. Roots greater than ½" around should be split before drying.

Feverfew: digestive aid, tonic, gas, bloating, migraine headaches, high blood pressure, and menstrual discomforts. (Parts used—leaves)

Growing Advice: plant root cuttings 18" apart, when temperatures reach 70 degrees. Partial shade. Compost. (Bees dislike it, so plant it where you don't want bees.)

Garlic: bacterial antibiotic, fungal antibiotic, parasitic antibiotic, protozoan antibiotic, antiseptic, food—poisoning treatment, high blood pressure, diabetes, high cholesterol, cancer prevention, bronchitis, urinary tract infection treatment, healing wounds, yeast infection. (Parts used—cloves)

Growing Advice: plant cloves 2" deep and 6" apart, in rich, deeply cultivated, and well—drained soil. Full sun. Cut back flower stalks during the summer.

Hops: antiseptic, digestive aid, sedative, insomnia, and toothache.

Growing Advice: plant root cuttings in hills 18" apart, in deeply cultivated, rich, moist soil. Full sun. Water often. Harvest female flowers in the fall, when they feel firm, turn amber colored, and are covered with yellow dust. Dry immediately. (Parts used—glandular hairs of the female fruits)

Hyssop: colds, flu, cough, cold sores, stimulant, aromatic, asthma, lungs, phlegm, sore throat, fever, stings, bites, kills body lice. (Parts used—leaves, flowers)

Growing Advice: plant seeds ¼" deep, 12" apart, in a dry, sunny location. Compost. Water seedlings every few days. Mature plants prefer less water. Once plants reach 18" high, and lose their aroma, cut back tops to promote leaf growth. Harvest leaves any time. Cut back entire plant to 4" above ground just before it flowers. (Parts used—leaves, flowers)

Juniper: anti—inflammatory, high blood pressure, arthritis, water retention, tonic, kidney/bladder troubles, helps prevent diseases, colds, and bronchitis. (Parts used—berries)

Growing Advice: Most juniper grows everywhere, and is of easy access.

Meadowsweet: bacterial antibiotic, anti—inflammatory, pain, food—poisoning treatment, fever, diarrhea, and arthritis. (Parts used—leaves, flower tops)

Growing Advice: plant root cuttings underground, in rich, moist, and well—drained soil, under partial shade. Harvest when in bloom.

Mints (spearmint/peppermint): stimulant, germicide, disinfectant, wounds, burns, scalds, insect bites and stings, eczema, hives, toothache, anesthetic, bacterial antibiotic, antiseptic, decongestant, digestive aid, healing wounds, tooth decay prevention, nausea, gas, morning sickness, menstrual cramps, pain, motion sickness, colds, cough, flu, head ache, fever, insomnia, heartburn, cold sores, food—poisoning treatment. (Parts used—leaves, flower tops)

Growing Advice: plant root cuttings (with node or joint) in rich, moist, and well—drained soil, under full sun, or partial shade. Cut back often. Cut back entire plant to just a few inches above ground when first flowers appear. Replant every 3 yrs.

Winter mint: bladder problems, gas, gonorrhea, stimulant, stomachache. (Parts used—leaves, flower tops)

Growing Advice: Plant root cuttings in rich, moist, well—drained soil. Full sun or partial shade. Trim frequently to prevent bushiness. Cut entire plant to a few inches above ground, when first flowers appear. Dig out and replant every few years.

Motherwort: tranquilizer, sedative, stress, insomnia, high blood pressure, and anxiety. (Parts used—leaves, flowers, stems)

Growing Advice: plant seeds 12" apart, in rich, moist, and well—drained soil. Full sun. Harvest entire plant after flowers bloom.

Mullein: asthma, lungs, bronchitis, cough, sore throat, (for lung afflictions, smoke), diarrhea, toothache, induce sleep, food poisoning treatment, hemorrhoids, relieve pain, remove warts, swollen joints, toothache, wash for open sores. (Parts used—leaves, flowers, roots)

Growing Advice: Plant seeds in light, sandy soil. Full sun. Harvest up to 1/3 of the leaves in the first year. Harvest the rest the following year, before flowers bloom. Pick flowers as they bloom. Self—sewer.

Passionflower: antiseptic, anxiety, burns, insomnia, pain, sedative, stress, tranquilizer, wounds. (Parts used—leaves)

Growing Advice: Plant seeds in rich, slightly acidic, well—watered, well—drained loam. Mostly sun, with partial shade. Can't handle temperatures below 15 degrees. Needs something to climb. Harvest the leaves when flowers bloom. Water well.

Pennyroyal: (don't use if pregnant) cough, cramps, decongestant, headache, itch, insect/snake bites, insect repellent, jaundice, mouth sores, nausea, phlegm, toothache, ulcers. (Parts used—leaves, flower tops)

Growing Advice: Plant root runner divisions in rich, well—watered, sandy, slightly acidic loam. Full sun. Cut entire plant to just a few inches above ground in the fall.

Red Clover: menopausal discomforts, blood purifier, wounds, menstruation discomforts. (Parts used—flower tops)

Growing Advice: Plant seeds in moist, well—drained soil (no gravel or sand). Harvest flowers when tops are in full bloom.

Rose: colds, flu. (Parts used—petals)

Growing Advice: Plant 2—yr—old, field grown budded stalk in an 18" deep trench, covered with loose soil. Full sun. Air circulation. Mulch. Cultivate 2 ft deep. ½ rotted manure, ½ humus. Let settle in trench for about 2 weeks before planting. Water well, in dry weather. Trim late in the day.

Rosehips: vitamin C, cold sores, use in teas for colds/flu. (Parts used—hips)

Growing Advice: Usually of easy access, in most areas…grows in most mountain regions.

Rosemary: tonic, stimulant, preservative.

Growing Advice: Plant cuttings in light, sandy, well—drained soil, leaving only 1/3 of each twig showing. Full sun. Don't over water. (Parts used—leaves)

Sage: antiperspirant, antiseptic, asthma, bronchitis, cold, cough, flu, food poisoning prevention, gas, headache, help grow hair (if there are still root follicles present), help stop bleeding, kidneys, liver, lungs, remove dandruff, sore throat, stomach ache, tonsillitis, tonic, stimulant, wounds, pneumonia, preservative. (Parts used—leaves)

Growing Advice: Plant root cuttings in well—drained soil. Full sun. Water well until fully established. Then, water less. Replace every few years. Mulch. Harvest leaves before buds open, by cutting entire plant down to 4" above ground.

White willow: headaches, pain, menstrual cramps, fever, etc. (Parts used—bark)

Growing Advice: (see Food>Nuts &Fruit section)

Yarrow: antiseptic, anxiety, bleeding, burns, chicken pox, diarrhea, diabetes, female/womb troubles, fever, gas, insomnia, tonic, increase circulation, menstrual discomforts, sedative, stress, tranquilizer, wounds. (Parts used—leaves, stems, flower tops)

Growing Advice: Plant seeds just under the surface of fine, well—drained, moderately rich soil. Keep moist until germination takes place (in about 2 weeks). 1 foot apart. Full sun. Harvest when in bloom.

Flowers

Chrysanthemum: maroon, purple, white/July—October.

Growing Advice: Divide root cuttings into small sections. Plant root cuttings in well—cultivated, rich, well—drained soil. Partial shade. Mulch. Compost. When plants have six leaves, pinch the tops. As each new branch develops six leaves, pinch the tops.

Daffodil

Growing Advice: Plant bulbs in September or October in well—cultivated soil, with compost, and well—rotted manure. Plant 6" deep and 6" apart in clumps. Pack well. Mulch. Remove mulch in early spring. Compost.

Geranium

Growing Advice: Plant seeds in December, 1/8" deep in fine soil. Keep moist until they germinate (in about two to three weeks). When seedlings have their first pair of true leaves, transplant to the garden. When plants have several leaves, pinch out growing tips. Keep in sunny, but cool location. Giving them a surrounding barrier should help them grow better.

Iris: all shades/June, and some in spring and fall.

Growing Advice: Make sure leaves on each plant are turned away from its neighbors. Full sun. When first leaves begin to die (droop), remove them.

Winter Jasmine: yellow

Growing Advice: Plant rootstalks in well—drained loam. Full sun.

Lavender: stimulant, aromatic, tonic

Growing Advice: Plant cuttings in dry, light, well—drained loam, 12—15" apart.

Lilac

Growing Advice: Set root cuttings in sand, under glass until they have taken root. In September, plant in the garden. Full sun. Well—drained, loamy soil. Compost. Mulch in late fall.

Tulip

Growing Advice: Plant bulbs (twist them into place) in deep, (between 6 and 9") rich, well—drained, light loam, between October and November. Compost. Partial shade.

Storage

Dry. Crush into small pieces, for teas. Grind into a fine powder, for salves.

Preparations

Tea—for medicinal purposes: (internal) 1 Tsp. dried herb, to 1 Cup boiling water. Pour 1 Cup boiling water over 1tsp dried herb, and let steep for 5—10 minutes. Use more herbs to make tea stronger. For medicinal purposes, drink 4 Cups/day (1 Cup before each meal, and 1 Cup before retiring.)

Salve—(external) 2 Cups ground /dried herb (aloe, sage, mint, dill, echinacea, meadowsweet, apple leaves, blackberry, rosemary, and yarrow; plus, any others you may wish to add) to 3 Cups nut oil, and 1/2 Cup beeswax; mix together, cover, and solar heat in the sun for about three or four hours. When it is cooled, it will be firm and ready for use. Store in dark, cool area, like a cellar.

Flowers: extract oils when fresh.

Note: Just as a general rule, make sure plants have plenty of winter protection, such as wind protection barriers, and mulch.

Tip: Use pine needles (among other acidic plants) to give acidity to the soil.

Compost in the spring, mid—summer, and fall.

Most of these plants should be planted in early spring, or by early summer—when temperatures reach 50—70 degrees.

To extract the oil of an herb, such as rose, mint, etc.

Gather the herb/flower, (fresh is better, but dried should work too), place in a pan with rain/spring water. Weigh the petals down with a strainer or glass dish. Let steam for at least 1—5 hours, or until oil stops floating to the top. (Do not boil). When the water is thick, it is ready. Separate the oil from the water, and store in bottles with a cork in the top. Store in a cellar.

To extract oils from say, nuts, seeds, or the like...use an oil press. Pressing the oils as much as possible preserves more nutrients...especially vitamin E, among other antioxidants. (Such as when nut oils are to be used in soaps, lotions, etc.)

Replant some flowers/plants every year, whether to make sure you have continuous crops, or simply to have that type of plant.

Dyes: berries, flowers, and herbs. (Have some fun; experiment.)

For makeup, paint, etc.: Dry, crush, and grind into fine powder. Mix with water until at correct thickness, and use.

For material: Boil the plant, strain, and soak material in the colored water.

Personal Hygiene

Floss

Instructions: Use homemade thread, soaked in mint oils, and beeswax. Keep them in a cool, dark place so the wax on the floss doesn't melt. You can be creative, and soak the thread in mint oils, along with the other herbs used for toothpaste. This will help get the nutrients to the tight cracks and spaces in the teeth.

Laundry detergent

Instructions: Use shampoo, and/or use screwed up batches of soap. Add red clover, and any other herbs you may wish to add. Just be sure to use the herb *oils* as much as possible, and that there are not any major chunks or pieces of herb in the mix.

Shampoo

Ingredients: 5 oz. grated soap, 30 oz. water, and 1/2 tsp of powdered pectin (to extract from apples: Use left—over, bruised, and/or green apples. Wash, trim, and cut into small pieces. Boil the apples in 2 cups water per pound of apple pieces, for 15 minutes. Separate and remove any juices by using a strainer or coffee filter, but don't squish out any pulp. Place the pulp back in the pot, and add the same amount of water again.

Now, let the mixture simmer for another 15 minutes, but turn down the heat a bit. Let the mixture set for about 10 minutes, and strain again. Squish out the remaining juice, sundry the pulp/pectin, and store in glass jars in a cellar.

Instructions: Combine the ingredients listed above, and heat the mixture until smooth, and liquid. Then, add several drops chamomile oil (for light hair) or rosemary oil (for dark hair), several drops of pine oil, and several drops of sage oil. Fill empty shampoo bottles. Shake well before use.

Additional ingredients: Berry juice, herb oils (like rosemary), or others listed in the Soap section below, under Additional ingredients. Aloe gel, Cantaloupe and Strawberry juices, Hyssop, Almond, sunflower seed, and sage oils, are definitely recommended.

Cantaloupe and Strawberries are high in Folic acid and Vitamin C.
Hyssop kills/prevents body lice.
Almond oil has minimal Vitamin A content, but is high in Vitamin **E**, B1, B2, B6, Protein, Biotin, and has some Folic Acid.
Sunflower Seed oil has minimal Vitamin E content, but is high in Vitamin **A**, B1, B2, B6, and Protein.
Sage is an antiperspirant, helps grow hair if there are any follicles left to grow them from, and will prevent dandruff.

Variations: Use equal parts Oat, and Barley Milk in place of water. They help thicken and add nutrients to the mixture, whether it is to be used for soap, shampoo, or just about anything. Barley milk can be made in the same way as oat milk, and is rich in folic acid.

Aloe Gel, Almond, and Sunflower seed oils all contain substantial amounts of Vitamin E, other antioxidants (like Vitamins A, and C), the B Vitamins (like B6, biotin, and folic acid), and plant proteins necessary for good, shiny, and healthy hair growth.

Soap

Basic Ingredients: Nut oil (almond oil), sunflower seeds, potash (banana skin is about 42% potash, and corncob ash—about 50%), aloe vera (squish into consistent gel), strawberry, sage, pennyroyal, dill, echinacea, meadowsweet, and mint oils.

Additional ingredients: Herbs (see Herbs), and flowers such as—Jasmine, lavender, lilac, pine, rose, geranium, tulip, chrysanthemum, daffodil, iris, etc.

Instructions: (Before using the nut oils, melt, and see if there is any separation. If there is, use the clear portion. If not, use it all.) Put on rubber gloves, and safety glasses. Slowly, pour cold water through a potash siv until potash mixture weighs 44 oz. minus the weight of the glass container, while stirring with a wooden spoon. (Avoid breathing in fumes). As soon as the potash is dissolved in the water, set it aside to cool. Weigh out 48 oz. Almond oil, and 38 oz. Brazil nut oil. Melt over low heat, stirring frequently. Get both the potash mixture and the oils to a temperature range of between 95 and 98 degrees. Use hot or cold water baths to raise or lower the temperature of the mixtures. (Make sure to stir each mixture before taking the temperature). Slowly, pour in and constantly stir a steady stream of potash mixture into the oils until it has all been combined. Stir for another 10 minutes, or until the mixture becomes thick enough to *begin* dribbling designs on the top of the soap mixture. Now is the time to add herb/flower oils, petals, seeds, oats, etc. (***Do it quick!***). Grease the inside of whatever molds you'll use with beeswax, or nut butter. Pour your mixture into the molds, and cover with a lid. Place in an undisturbed, warm place and cover with several layers of thick blankets. Let sit for 18 hours to complete the saponification process. Remove the blankets and lid. Leave the soap where it is for another 8—12 hours before removing from the molds. To make sure the soap has completed the saponification process, touch a bar of soap to your tongue. If the soap sort of burns your tongue, it isn't done. (If it isn't done, you can cover the soap with boiling water, let it jellify, and use it for laundry soap.) To make soap on a rope, just fill the molds halfway, tie the ends of a small rope together, place the rope on top of the soap—to—be, (with the tied ends toward the inside), and fill the molds the rest of the way. Finish making the soap with the same directions as above.

Removing hair

Instructions: heat beeswax up to about 100 degrees or so, and apply to legs, or area where you want to remove hair. Let cool/dry; peal off really fast. Ouch! But it works.

Rabbit Skin Moccasins

Instructions: (would be very warm and comfortable/flexible). Just trace around your feet on a piece of fur (with skin still attached, and tanned); give room for, and stitch them up the sides.

SHELTER

Note: If you have any questions or comments, you are welcome to e—mail me at any time. I strongly recommend that you go to your local bookstore, or get online and buy *The Cob Builder's Handbook*, by Becky Bee, before starting your house—building project. There are many helpful hints, tips, and specifications, which may prove to be very useful in guiding you through a project of this proportion. If you were real nice, I might even research subjects if you really want more information, but don't have the time, or know where to look.

claudiac@highdesertnet.com

Floor Plan/Blueprint: First, you need to ask yourself some questions, such as the following:

- What style, do I like best? Victorian? French? Spanish? Bright, and open, with high ceilings? Closed in and cozy?
- How many people will be residing in the home? How many bedrooms will we need? Bathrooms? How much over—all space do we need? How many floors do I want, and will everyone in the home have access to them?
- What are my favorite colors/schemes? How will they fit in with the overall design of the home?
- What kind of *feel* do I want when I walk in? (Remember, this will be your home, and you want the opportunity of taking pride in doing things right the first time, instead of wasting a lot of time and money just to have to do it all over again. Besides, if you have

to do it all over, you might kill the mood, to do it right the second time).

Finish this process, by creating in your mind, how many rooms you want, and where. Then, draw it out on graph paper, and start walking through the house in your mind. Imagine every little detail down to where you want your sinks, tubs, walls, nooks, shelves, built—in furniture/accessories, inlets and outlets, power room for electrical features, everything. Draw it all out on paper. Know your exact coordinates for every wall, room, etc. Account for width of walls. (Walls will be about 2—3 feet wide at the bottom, so take into account an extra 3 feet or so in wall width).

Preparation: First, tap plenty of pine trees, or other pitch producing trees, like you would with maple trees. Hang buckets from the taps in early spring, and at the end of the summer, take the buckets of pitch, and pour them all into several medium sized, or one, big cast iron pot. (The old kind you can hang from a tri—pod above a fire outside).

Once the trees are tapped, all you can do is wait…so in the meantime, purchase a small saw mill to use for cutting trees and lumber.

(**Note:** Make sure you know about the building codes and permits necessary in your area, and regarding your land, before starting any construction project involving your safety, and legality). This type of half—chainsaw, half sawmill, is not very expensive. The average price for something like this is only about $300—1,500. Just look in the classifieds in the ***Mother Earth Magazine.*** They have a lot of helpful hints on many subjects of this sort. They even have a website at *www.motherearthnews.com*. Also, *www.earthship.com* has information regarding building codes.

You should know how much lumber you will need for the roof, door-frames, floors, window frames, roof beams, support beams, what size of lumber you will need, etc. Once you have determined the sizes and amount of lumber you will need: cut, peel, and prepare boards, beams, and frames. They will need to stay dry for a year more or less to help cure, so lay them layer by layer, between crates, so they don't rot by lying on the ground, or not getting enough air. Cover them with tarps, to keep rain, snow, and moisture out.

Now that you have your lumber, your sap, your floor plan, your blueprint, etc…where will you want your house to be? First of all, you should know which direction your water sources will come from, and where gray water will exit. Find a SE, SW, or southern slope. This will help by:

- Maximizing sunlight in the winter
- Helping to regulate temperatures inside
- Keeping exterior water temperatures from freezing before entering the cistern
- Helping to prevent pipes from freezing, breaking, or needing replacement
- Requiring less maintenance

Once you find the location, stake out every exterior corner, taking in account the width of the walls. Then tie, and run a string from one stake to the next, to give you an outline, as to the shape of foundation you will need.

Foundation

Dig a hole, in the shape of your floor plan outline, about 3 feet deep, depending on how much weight will be resting on the foundation. Make sure the interior floor and sides of the foundation are level. Now, heat up the pitch in the pot, above a fire outside. Get it warm enough to be pliable, but not hot enough to boil. Spread a thick layer of pitch along floor, and all sides of the interior of the foundation. Let cool, and harden. Fill the foundation with cob (pitch in the mix) and rocks, packing firmly as you progress. Build this cob/rock wall foundation up to about 3 feet above ground. (This would be 6 feet high, from 3 feet underground, to 3 feet above ground...ample stability/strength, even for two levels).

Rock/Cob Foundation

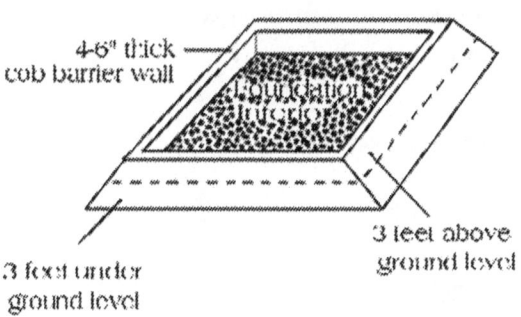

4-6" thick cob barrier wall

Foundation Interior

3 feet above ground level

3 feet under ground level

Before allowing the exterior portion (above ground) of the foundation to dry, squish in gravel on the outside, leaving very little space between the tiny rocks. Shingles are made this way; only they are made with tarred building paper, instead of cob/pitch. Long before my time, boats were sealed with pitch. Cob is fire proof, and pitch is waterproof. When mixed together, they compliment one another.

Remember to firmly pack down the rock/cob wall as you build it, making sure all is level. Once finished with the structure, compact it again. One way to do this is to use one of your (stripped and peeled) logs to roll it out like dough. On the outer most edge of the floor of the foundation, create a small barrier wall out of the cob mixture. This should look like a frame, and be about 6 inches high by 6 inches wide.

Plumbing

Assuming that you have already built the cistern, any other feeding streams to it, and have successfully installed the water lines all the way to about 10 feet from the house: (Dig 3 foot deep trenches to bury the pipes; pack the pipes in straw, and cover with dirt.)

Start with marking the particular positions on the foundation in which the water will be coming in, (such as the initial entrance, the kitchen sink, bathrooms, etc.), and where the gray water will be diverted to/exit from.

Solar Water Heaters

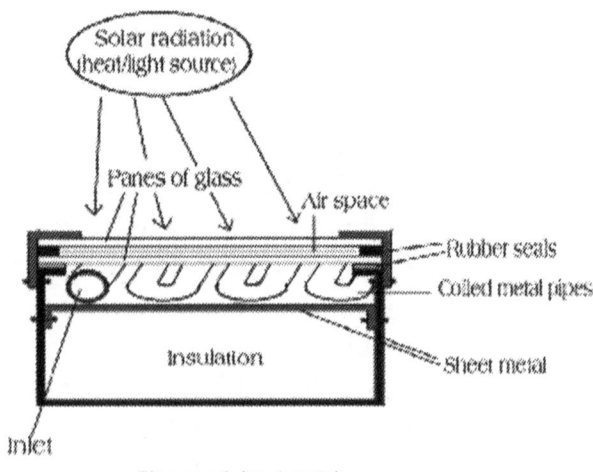

To build the solar collector/s, create a box made from sheet metal, which is totally sealed, (water proof), and insulated in the bottom two thirds portion of the box. Paint all exposed sides of the box flat black, and allow the paint to dry. This will be the casing. (Note: you can make the casing with two metal boxes, just like the solar cooker, for an even better design). You will also need a square piece of sheet metal cut into the same shape as the casing, which has been painted flat black on both sides, with non—water soluble, latex/waterproof paint. (The paint should be able to withstand temperatures up to 300 degrees as well…possibly 400 degrees).

Hold this above the insulation with L brackets, rivets, and felt strips to help seal, and to keep it from moving out of position. The pipes holding the water that is to be heated, should follow a coiled path, and be placed on top of the flat, black sheet metal.

About ½ to one inch above the pipes should be two glass panes…each separated by ½ to one inch. All should be completely water/air tight, and of course, the collector needs openings for entrances and exits, which are also sealed. Apply insulation tape, and felt between glass and metal. Collector should be above ground, facing South, SW, or SE, and at a 30 to 45 degree angle. If you want hot water by noon, face SE; if you want hot water after noon, face SW.

There should be 1—1 ½ square feet collector area, per gallon of water you want to heat.

Can be one big collector, or, preferably, several collectors interconnected, and combined to flow through one final solar water heater. This will make it easier to adjust the direction the collector/s faces, if or whenever it may be necessary.

Can install up to four reflector lids to concentrate heat and light energy from the sun.

Pipes should be metal, painted flat black on the outside, and about 1" around per 30 feet total collector size.

Water Purification

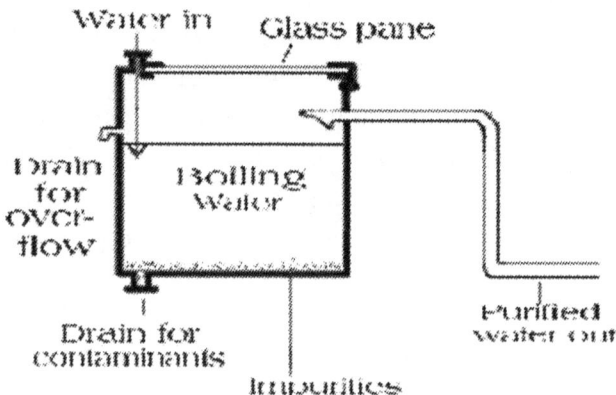

First, your water would come *down* from a cistern (as shown in "the basic overall system"), into the solar hot water heaters. Then, you would divert the water from the water heaters, through the water distiller. (Shown to your above).

Water would flow through yet one more, and final solar water heater, to keep it close to boiling level. (This final solar hot water heater should be as close to the home as possible).

Then, hot water lines would flow in the shape of a coil under the floors, thereby radiating heat from below, *and* purifying your water at the same time.

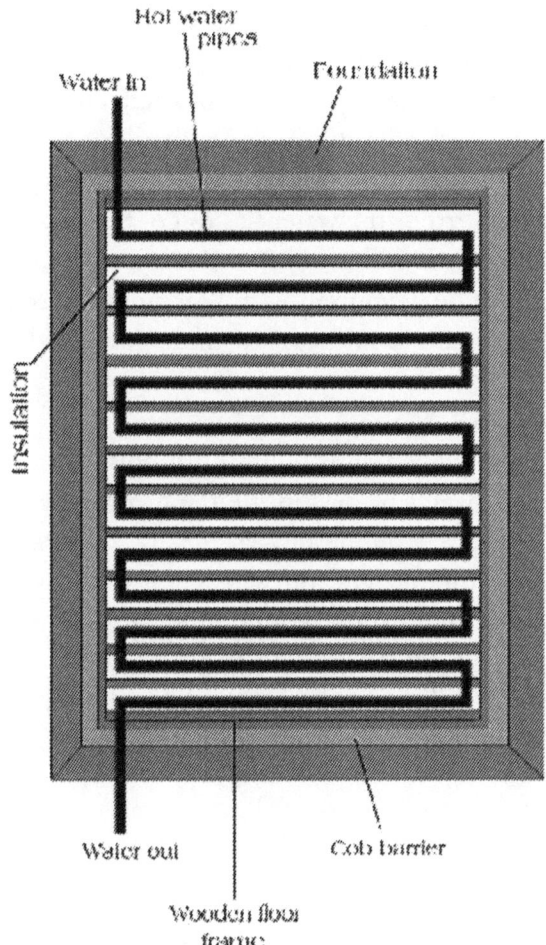

You will need to have access to all plumbing. Clean out water heaters/distiller as often as necessary. To add to the flow of water, you may want to install rain gutters around the bottom of all eaves of the roof of the home. Apply 1/8 to ¼ inch fine wire mesh screen to the top of all gutters, and cistern entrances. Then lead all the gutters to the same pipe, which will lead water to the 2nd cistern, or to places in need of irrigation…such as the greenhouse/s.

Distillation is one of the easiest, and most effective ways of removing contaminates from untreated water, and by coiling the hot water under the floors, one is providing more energy efficiency to the home. Remember that the further the water has to go, the cooler it will get. The less distance, the hotter it will be.

You won't want to burn yourself with boiling water, so be sure to allow for enough travel time to cool it off to more comfortable temperatures, before reaching the faucets.

Note: You might want to include a greenhouse/s in the design, and place your solar hot water heaters inside the greenhouse/s. This way, you have hot water all year—round, and can separate hot water lines, so hot water in one area won't depend on whether it is being used in another area. You know how when you're taking a shower, someone uses water in the kitchen, and you get burned or froze? Including a medium sized greenhouse on the North and East sides of the home, installing more solar water heaters, and separating hot water lines will prevent this from happening.

Cold Water

All the water will be naturally distilled, before entering the home, by means of boiling, and condensing. Therefore, the water would first be hot, before it could be cold…so you would have to cool off the water. This can create a problem, because you don't want your cold water to be hot, or vise versa, you wouldn't want cold water flowing under the floors, (that would defeat the purpose of coiling your hot water lines under the floors to add heat), and you can't let them freeze. One way to solve this is to divide the directions of hot and cold pipes…hot water would flow through coiled pipes under the floors. Cold water would go around the exterior of the house, about three to four feet underground. This would keep temperatures for the cold water lines at about 60 degrees. The further you divert the cold water lines, the cooler they will get. (They will not likely get cooler than maybe 55 degrees all year round, if you fill the trenches with straw, or other insulator before covering the pipes with dirt).

Floor on First Level

Within the outer cob frame of the foundation, build a large wooden frame with 2 x 4's, which touches all edges of the interior of the cob frame. Then, screw down more boards within the frame, so it would look like shelves lying down. Fill the frame about half way up with straw or other insulation, and place pipes on top of the insulation. Connect all plumbing, and make sure all is working properly. If all is running smooth, fill the frames (covering the pipes) the rest of the way with insulation.

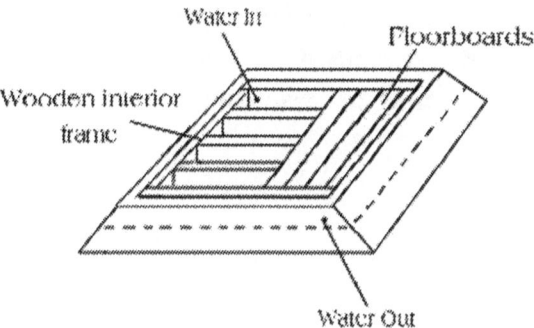

Screw your floorboards *across* the top of the frame on the foundation. Even if you screw the floorboards down, they shouldn't be hard to remove, so no one would have to go outside and crawl under the house to get to the pipes.

Once the floorboards are installed, (and in the process of interior decorating), you can either polish them for wooden floors, cover the wooden floors with carpet, or install a rock floor. You could also incorporate the use of all of these methods.

To Build a Rock Floor

Cover the floorboards with chicken wire. Nail it down. Then apply a 4—6 inch layer of cob, with rock slabs or slate squished in and caulked between. (The rock slabs should be level with the caulking). Make sure all is level before allowing it to dry. It would be harder to access the plumbing, but it can be done.

Structural Walls

Now that you have your floor, you can start building your structural walls. Walls can be built simply by plopping gobs of cob (mixture of clay, sand, and straw) in mounds, and forming the walls with your hands, a board, and a level, as it ascends. Cob is as strong as concrete or bricks, when dry. It is moldable, highly insulative, and needs no forms, support beams, or rebar.

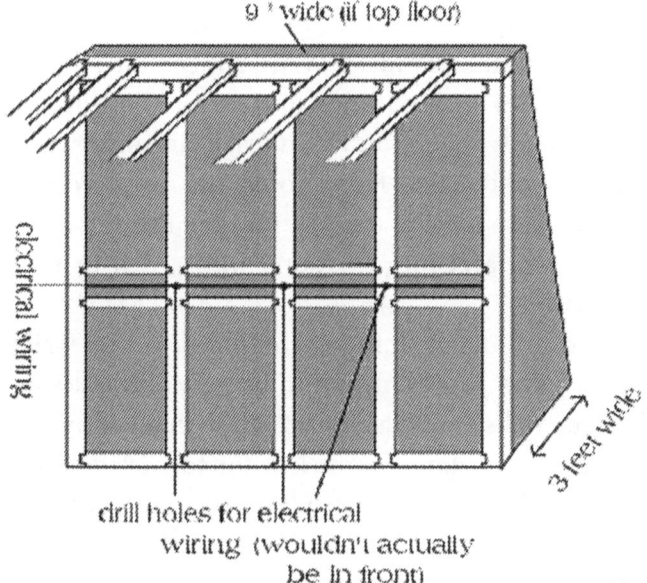

9 ' wide (if top floor)

electrical wiring

3 feet wide

drill holes for electrical
wiring (wouldn't actually
be in front)

Note: gray colored areas represent cob

Typically, with cob designs, the width of the walls starting from the floor up, should be about two to three feet wide, tapering up to no less than 9 at the top of the wall/s. (The foundation wall would follow the same tapering angle).

Remember to leave room for future electrical wiring, and their housings within the walls.

Also, build in a wooden frame with support beams, all the way around the interior of the outer most walls. There should be beams or cob pillars standing about five to eight feet apart, with support beams lying on top, underneath, and between the vertical support beams. You can still cover the beams with cob so it all looks the same, but you'll have to apply chicken wire for the cob to hang on to. After all beams are connected, they should look like a row of square frames. I know, cob walls do not need support, but the floors above will need some extra support, and so will the roof, (especially if you plan on having more than one level).

For the exterior portion of outside walls, apply a thick layer of cob with pitch and cattail fuzzies or sifted straw in the mix. (For the small pieces of straw, you can take a wooden frame, and nail on some wire mesh; then place straw inside, and shake. Keep doing this until you have enough screened straw to add to the cob mixture for the outside walls. This is your plaster mix). Squish gravel into the outer most, inch or two of exterior walls before cob dries.

Build the interior walls the same as you did the outer walls, only don't squish in gravel (unless you want that to be part of the design). The bottom of the interior walls would also start out with a width of about 2 to 3 feet thick, tapering up to about 9" thick at the top. Make sure all walls are level on the tops (and tapered on the sides), according to the height of the second floor.

Leave doorways and hallways open, adding rock arches or wooden frames for them as you build.

(**Note:** Remember to build in shelves, coves, furniture, or other built—in features, such as electrical wiring and their housings before allowing walls to dry).

Second Floor (if there is one)

Place and secure support beams or logs horizontally, going from the outer to the inner walls. Leave about 5—8 feet between them, staggering their weight to the middles of the vertical beams. (To get an idea as to what this should look like, refer to the previous picture of an exterior wall).

Next, *lay your 5—8 foot long, 3—inch thick, strong* floorboards across the top of these beams/logs, from left to right, (or vise versa) fitting them together real tight. Screw the floorboards down, and finish floors with the same methods used for the first floor.

Be sure to build yourself a strong rail to hold on to, along any open loft line edges, so no one will fall over, and of course, build the stairs to get up there.

Stairs can be built the same as the walls, molding cob as you ascend, and adding built—in features as you build them.

Remember to make sure the tops of the walls above the second floor are level with the angle of the roof.

Roof

You will need those support beams again. Using the beams, (2 x 4s, or 4 x 6s) build frames in the shape of an "A", all the way across the length and width of the outside walls. There should be about five to eight feet of space between each frame, with one being on each end. Each frame should also be connected to the next, making one big roof frame. Add another foot, more or less, to the outside of the frame, for an overhang. If you want skylights, integrate them within the design of the roof frame as you build. The peak of the roof should generally be at the center of the home, and situated at an average of a 30 to 45 degree angle above walls. After installing and connecting the frames for the roof, cover the interior roof (ceiling) with board ends or floorboards. Build the window frames in as you progress. Seal, and fill in the outside portion of the roof with cob (mix in a little pitch, and some sifted straw). In the furthest layer of cob to the outside, squish in as much small gravel as you can. Let dry completely. For the ceiling inside, apply chicken wire, or something for the cob to hold onto. Plaster the ceiling (and walls, inside and out) with your cob plaster mix.

For a plaster mix, shake the straw through ¼" wire mesh screen, and/or add some cattail fuzzies to the cob mix. After drying, you can paint the inside/outside of the home with a latex, waterproof paint.

Once the roof is finished, install the glass for any skylights that may be a part of the design.

Bathrooms and Kitchens

Toilets and sinks usually come with instructions on how to install them. Using waterless/odorless compost toilets will greatly reduce the amount of water your family uses, and eliminate the need for DEQ approvals, septic, sewage, drain field, black water problems/treatment, etc.

For a nice tub, you can find a tub liner you really like, and take its measurements. Then, using the measurements, build a tub with cob, into the floor.

On the top few inches of the cob tub molding, leave it with a rough surface. Let the form dry completely. Paste a 2" thick layer of cob (with a little pitch in the mix) on the inside of the tub mold, and push the liner down into it. Squish the liner into the tub mold really tight, pushing out any air bubbles you might find. You'll want to cut off any excess cob, which has been squished out. Trim the outsides where cob and liner come together, like you would a pie.

For the walls inside the shower/tub, build a rock wall using the same method as you would for a rock floor.

Counters for sinks or the kitchen, can be molded with cob and rocks too.

Power

A hybrid combination solar/wind—powered system is the best choice for someone living off—grid. The place you buy this from can help inform you on how to install what you can, what portions of the process has to be overseen or performed by electricians, and about the building codes to watch out for. They can help you determine the size of system you will need, based on your average energy consumption. A place to visit, offering good prices/packages on solar/wind systems, is *www.fords-mtm.com*. Have a qualified electrician install these systems for you, if you don't know what you are doing. (Make sure to include a power control room in your floor plan, before you start building).

Water

Again, *www.earthship.com* is also a good resource to find the best prices, systems, and services. They can help you design, and build a water purification system, water pressure system/regulation, cistern package, and provide you with all other services/products, that are right for your family. They can help you design virtually every aspect of your new home, using the same general materials as shown in this chapter.

Heat

A backup heat source is something you'll want to include in your design, not necessarily because you'll need it, but because of building codes. Your home will most likely stay at an average constant temperature of 60—70 degrees, all year around anyway. How? Because earth is a very good insulator, and because tilted windows at the angle of the roof (skylights) will naturally soak up maximum solar radiation (heat) in the winter, and minimum heat in the summer. You can install a cast iron wood stove, or build a cob fireplace within the structure of the walls. Earthen fireplaces are excellent heat sources! And, you can sculpt them into just about any form you want.

To distribute heat evenly to particular portions of the home, you can build an addition to the backside of the fireplace, which is completely closed in, and made with cob, so it is fire proof. Divert the stovepipe not straight up through the roof, like most homes, but first through the addition behind the stove/fireplace. Leave a hole at the bottom of the addition, big enough for a fan to pull/force the hot air through heating ducts, which are lead to wherever you want them. To make the hole the right size for the chosen fan, place a coffee can, or something similar, in the place where the fan will be; take the can out after the cob dries enough to keep the shape, but before it dries completely. Make sure air leaks are limited, and build everything into the structure of the walls as you build the home. After leading the stovepipe through the addition, let the smoke rise up and escape from the stovepipe through the roof. This, I call the non—electric forced air—heating system. (Though, you still need electricity to use the fan, the electricity used is minute compared to the electricity used with heating elements in the typical forced air heating system). To help minimize energy consumption, install a wood stove *within* the structure of the cob fireplace, but don't cover the back of the stove with cob; leave space between the back of the stove and the backside of the addition. This will radiate more heat through the back of the stove into the addition, and will help keep excess heat from escaping out the front and sides.

If you include a greenhouse in your floor plan, or one on the North and East sides of your home, (they don't have to be very large; 20 feet squared, is fine), it will help increase the average year—round temperature of your home to about 70—75 degrees, and provide you with more oxygen and fresh air. It will also help the solar hot water heaters do their job in providing hot, and clean water all year around.

So, now you are using direct energy from the sun to heat and purify your water, hot water to heat floors, the hot air from a stovepipe to heat the walls and air inside, and the greenhouse/s to heat and protect portions of the outside of the home from cold winds. And, of course, we all know that hot air and water rises, and since all heat will be forced to come from below, it will rise, and be of better use.

Light

You can use electric lighting, but in case you want or need the use of candles, here's how to make them:

Braid strings together, which end up being about ½ centimeter around, more or less after braided. Take a metal ring with a circumference of about 3" around or more; tie three strings, opposite of each other, on what will be the top of the ring. Go up from there about 3 or 4". Tie these strings into one. (This will be what you hold on to in the process of dipping the wicks; you can also build a frame to hold several of these rings, so you can make a bunch of candles at once). Tie the tops of the wicks to the bottom side of the ring/s, spacing them apart at least ½ inch. Melt beeswax, and strain. If you want plain candles, use as is. If you want scented or colored candles, now is the time to add the desired aromatic herb oils, dyes, and/or flower petals, oats, etc. to the melted wax. Now, dip the wicks into the wax bath, leaving the wicks in for a few seconds each time. Then lift them up and out of the wax vat, keeping them level with each other. (Keep the wax mix at melting point until you are done). Repeat this process, over and over again, until candles are at the desired thickness. You can also manipulate the shape of the candles, by dipping only the desired portions of the candles in the wax bath. The more you dip, the bigger that part of the candle will be. Once you achieve the basic shape of the candle/s, you can cut them into yet another design.

Humidity

Make sure to leave some vents in various places, leading from a lower level outside, and up through the walls/roof. Have openings in places easy to reach. You should do this, so you don't get excess humidity, and water condensation on the walls. If you don't, you could have rain inside! Or, because your walls are made of cob, excess condensation could not only weaken the walls, but the walls would more than likely soak up the water, and expand. Then, eventually, the water would evaporate with heat, the walls would dry, and then they would shrink. In the shrinking process, they might crack. If this process goes on, on a regular basis, it wouldn't take too long before the walls would eventually just collapse.

Cellar

As a matter of comfort, build the cellar as a part of the house so you can get there without having to go outside, but make sure you close it off so the temperature in the cellar is cooler than that of the home. To build the structure, start with a foundation, the same as with the house. Instead of building the exterior walls with cob, create a rock wall, by lining and stacking rocks in rows on top of each other, and pulling dirt in behind them.

Keep doing this from the bottom to the top row of rocks, until the walls are about 8—10 feet high. Make sure all is as level as possible. (You can dig the foundation a few feet deeper, so the cellar will only be a few more feet above ground level). At this point, you should make sure the walls are bermed with earth to the highest row of rocks. Build the roof the same as you did for the house, only you won't need windows. Apply an extra layer of pitch on the inside and outside of the roof, and the inside of the rock walls to seal. Build the floor, ceiling, and interior walls with cob, (and floorboards), the same as with the home. Finally, cover the rest of the structure, except any exits you may want to the outside, with at least one to four feet of earth. Remember to build in arch doorways as you go. To help prevent erosion, plant grass (or any plants that don't need a whole lot of room for the roots) in the soil sitting on the roof of the cellar.

The only thing left, is for your imagination to take over, and decorate the interior of your new home with furniture, closets, personal items that make it home to you and your family, and the like.

A Note About Water and Electricity

Refrigerators, electric forced air heating systems, dryers, washers, dish-washers, and cooking stoves consume massive amounts of electricity and/or water. The more water/electricity you use, the more time and money you will spend on a cistern, and solar/wind electrical system.

For this reason, I have included the paragraphs below, to give you ideas on how you can save energy and water.

Refrigerators

Build a cellar to help preserve foods. If you rely on the foods in the Food chapter, you should have no trouble with preservation. Dry the fruit, bake—dry oats and barley, make granola with the nuts, seeds, barley, oats, and honey; dry the herbs; freeze—dry berries, can the juices; prepare the foods/herbs immediately after harvesting. Store in the cellar.

The main foods that require refrigeration are the berries, comfrey, and other foods containing antioxidants, such as Vitamins A, C, and E. These vitamins are destroyed by light, heat, and oxidation. I would suggest get-ting a 20 cubic foot freezer, and a home freeze—dryer. You would freeze the food/herb first, and freeze—dry them once frozen. Then, you could store everything in the cellar. It shouldn't take too much electricity, com-pared to a refrigerator, because you wouldn't have to use the freezer all year around. If you wanted, you could also use a small refrigerator for goodies, juice, iced tea, etc.

Electrical Forced Air Heating Systems

Described earlier in this chapter, under "Heat".

Dryers

You can easily use the greenhouse/s to dry your clothes on clotheslines, all year around. Just be sure to have vents to prevent excessive humidity, and mildew. You can also lead one or more of the heating ducts to a spot underneath clotheslines, to help heat and dry them faster.

Washers

You can have an electric washer if you want, but be warned; washers use a lot of electricity, and waste water. You can build a home washing area with cob, just like you did for the tubs/showers, but build it bigger. (Or you can design your tub to be used as a tub, shower, and clothes washing area). Washing clothes by hand really isn't very hard, and doesn't take much longer than a washing machine; use a washboard at an angle at the edges of the washing tub to wash out stains. Just be sure to build your washing tub so that you won't have to sit or kneel in uncomfortable positions…you don't want to have a sore back. You might also want to wear some thin gloves, to keep the skin on your hands from rubbing themselves raw, if you have a ton of laundry to do at one time.

There are also basic instructions to make your own laundry detergent in the Personal Hygiene section.

Dishwashers

Dishwashers are for the lazy; and besides, what's the point? You still have to wash the dishes before you wash them in the dishwasher. What a waste of time, water, and electricity.

Cooking Stoves

You can build a solar cooker, by welding sheet metal into the shape of two boxes; one box will be placed inside the other. The outer box should be about ½ to 1" larger all the way around, so there is air space between them. The larger box should also be at least 1—2" taller than the smaller box. Decide how big you want your solar cooker to be, by first deciding how many pots/pans you want to be able to use at one time, and by averaging out the size of the largest pot or pan you will be using to cook with. (This can also be used in baking). The larger box should reach about one inch above where the top of your largest pot or pan will be.

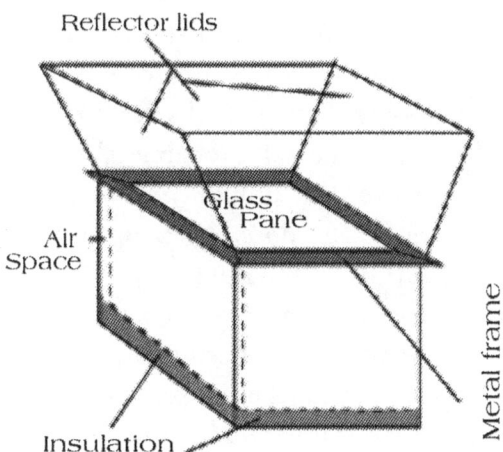

Paint both boxes flat black with anodized, non—toxic, waterproof, fireproof paint.

On the top of the outer box, weld three—inch wide strips of metal into a frame on all sides. (If your air space is to be one inch wide, and your strips are three inches wide: place the metal strips with a 2" overhang to the outside, and one inch to the inside.)

This will be the frame to hold the smaller box in place. Place some straw, or a small cattail fuzzy pillow in the bottom of the larger box, and wrap ten—foil all the way around it…this will serve as insulation, and should be thick enough (about 1"), so that when you place the smaller box inside the larger one, the tops of both boxes are level with each other. There should be very little, if any air space between insulation and the inside walls in the bottom portion of the cooker box. Now, place the smaller metal box on top of the insulation pillow, inside of the larger metal box. Weld the tops of the boxes together, and paint the inside of the inner box with another coat of flat black paint. Allow the paint to dry. Now that you have your base, cut four more pieces of sheet metal the same size as the base of the solar cooker. (These will be the reflector lids). Use hinges that only open to an angle of about 30—40 degrees, to connect the bottoms of the reflector lids to the top of the base. Glue aluminum foil on the underside of the reflector lids, and place a (removable) pane of glass on top of the base of the solar cooker. This style of solar cooker should get up to about 300 degrees. Cooking time will probably take almost twice as long as a conventional oven/stove, but unlike conventional ovens, the solar cooker requires no electricity, and doesn't heat up the rest of the kitchen. No more sweatin' your butt off over a hot stove!

You can build this into your counter top, (making sure it receives ample sunlight), or take it out whenever you need it, and place/take it anywhere you want. Just remember that the solar cooker does not require electricity to be running, so if you build it into your counter top, you should be able to close the reflector lids, to keep it from cooking all day.

Some Interior additions

Braided Rugs: Take material from just about any cloth/clothes, from the thrift shop, or old clothes you don't need any more. Strip the material length—wise, into strips about 2" wide. Braid with two other strips into one, making one long, braided piece of rope.

Using a needle and thread, sew the braided rope around itself. (When you sew, you should keep the stitches on the inside, and between the braided ropes...don't wrap the ropes with string, you want the material to show). The bigger you want the rug to be, the more braided ropes you add. The shape you want, (such as a circle, or an oval), is not very hard to make. Just decide how round, or long you want your circle to be; the longer you make the interior, the longer (more oval) the outside will be.

Cattail fuzzy blankets: If you have, and know how to use a spinning wheel, and weaving loom...excellent! You can use cattail fuzzies like you would cotton, in the making of string, material, and for the use of stuffing. You can also use other plant fibers (the insides of the stalks) such as the inside of tree bark, cattail stalks, nettle, etc.

Once you have your material, cut out the pattern for the blanket top and bottom, leaving extra room for sewing double stitches. Lay the top and bottom sides of the blanket—to—be with the outsides in. Double stitch three sides of the top and bottom together with a sewing machine, or by hand.

For the inside, you can either use several worn out/used blankets, or stuff with cattail fuzzies. Whether you decide to stuff the blanket with more blankets, or with cattail fuzzies, make pockets by sewing vertical and horizontal lines, crossing each other, on the interior portion, every few inches to hold smaller portions of stuffing/blankets in place. (If you are using cotton, or cattail fuzzies to stuff your blanket, you will want to stuff as you sew the pockets and use two sets of top and bottom blankets). This will keep the blanket from wadding up in a ball, especially when washing.

Finally, turn the blanket right side out, finish sewing together the top and bottom of the blanket, (with the stuffing in between), leaving the extra material (edges) on the inside. Sew one or two more times all the way around the outer edge of the blanket, to connect the outer edges of the inner stuffing and the outside of the blanket together; or you can just sew a button on all corners. You can always make a blanket cover, just like you would for a pillowcase, if you want the same blanket, but with an option as to the look or feel of it from one day to the next.

Benefits of a Cob Home

With a house made from cob, pitch, and rocks, (preferably with virtually no air leaks), you shouldn't have any worries of rodents, insects, mice, termites, ants, or their families infesting and taking over your home. But just to be sure, dilute mint oil in water, (1 part mint oil to 2 parts water) and fill up a spray bottle. Spray this around every door or window that leads to the outside. This will stop insects from coming in through windows and doors. You can also use this to mop your floors with, as mints are also disinfectants.

Install screen windows and doors for when you want to leave them open, but don't want flies coming in.

Note: The main purpose for this section was to give ideas on how to build a house that is generally pest free, strong, and energy efficient. So many homes today are carelessly thrown together as fast as possible...today's home construction crews are more interested in quantity, than quality. The faster homes are built, the more money they make. The more time they take in doing that, the less money they make.

Walls in and around the average home are just a few inches (at the most) thick, and are to some extent, just plain flimsy. The R—value of the average home is only between 20 and 45%, whereas the cob home has an

R—value of about 99%! The walls in a cob home are between 9" and 3 feet thick, and are very strong.

People deserve a home with walls that won't shake, no matter how much or how far the washing machine bounces…walls that can't be punched, kicked, or ran through! Now *that's* a home you can count on lasting through generation after generation. Your home should be water and fire proof, and one that isn't going to be carried away by strong winds or heavy rains. And to top it all off, we should have homes that don't cost a fortune to build, heat, maintain, and insure!

Section 2:
Mental Health

Mental health is equally as important as physical health. For, the *state* of the mind is what determines the state of one's physical and spiritual bodies. The *condition* the state of the mind is in can be the gap, or it can be the bridge between mental and spiritual satisfaction. What you choose to see is what you get. The reality of your life is what you perceive it to be.

Though you may perceive the color of the sky to be blue, who is to say that what you are really seeing isn't red? Or green? Or purple? You call it "blue" because that is the word you were taught to use, in order to express that color; and in reality, the sky contains just as much purple as it does blue, and is therefore violet. We humans just don't have the physically fine tuned perceptual ability to see the true color of the sky and atmosphere.

Like produces like and yet, opposites attract

We all naturally push ourselves out, with our own, unique perceptions and identities...we all have a message to tell, and we all have a talent, which is meant to be used in servicing ourselves and others. Our own face of the divine shines through. Our true colors always come out. Like an ocean of glass; reflective, yet translucent, we become mirrors of what lies deep within the mind…our children become expressions of us, and what we do, as do we become expressions of the mind, and where it leads us.

We are but projections of our minds…what we know to be real and true, has manifested itself into our lives as a result of the knowledge contained within the prismatic spectrum of collective thought.

After thinking and believing the same things for so long: thoughts can become ideas, ideas can become goals, goals can be achieved, and all can become a reality.

Anything that can be created in the mind, and any thought held long enough can become real. It doesn't take a whole lot of force to send thoughts into progression, when concerned with universal laws and how the universe reacts to the slightest movement…including a change in human consciousness.

Each state of conscious is a different body…a different perspective. When white light merges with a prism, it is divided, and the "true colors come out"…the colors of the rainbow, and the energy vibration of the seven chakras appear. When the seven chakras, or colors, or tones of energy vibrations unite, we get a whole new beginning…a whole new color, tone, vibration, or variance of light. When all becomes one *again*, it is as the same as it was before, only the energy has entered into a new and higher frequency.

To give you a better idea, imagine you are playing an instrument, or even singing a song. There are eight keys in one octave. An octave is the pitch, or tone of a sound. (Frequency). The musical scale is as follows: c, d, e, f, g, a, b, c. Notice that when you start at c, you also end at c, and begin a whole new frequency of energy.

In the same way, chakra energy centers, the colors of a rainbow, any type of energy in my view, will always return to where they came, with the only difference being that of the frequency or tone…which is generally higher.

If you start with a blank piece of paper, you have nothing on it. It is white. (Absence of color). If you were to color a red line, then orange, then yellow, green, blue, indigo, and then violet…what do you have? Well, a piece of paper with seven different colored lines on it. So when you blend all the colors together, you have a black piece of paper. Note that white is the *absence* of color. Black is all the colors coming together to form a new color. White is the opposite of black, and yet, without one, there wouldn't be the other. In this way, they are attracted to one another, just as the positive end of a magnet is attracted to the negative end of another magnet.

This new color, black, is All and None, all in one…though it only took seven steps to get there, it requires all of these steps to become one final reality. (Which is the eighth).

The first step is the beginning, white, with nothing, emptiness, void (just as the void mentioned among scientists concerning the "invisible dark energy", which as of yet, cannot be measured because it is timeless, formless, and endless); the steps in the middle are the individual colors projected from their origin, and the last step is the end, black, all the colors combined into one, the completion of the circle.

White and black are two very good examples of opposites that are the same, which depend on each other to exist.

Now, even though I mentioned "the dark energy" in relation to white, note that white and black are one and the same, and yet they are exact opposites.

Introduction to TM

Transcendental Meditation, (TM) is a way, or a mental path, if you will…to the bridge of your subconscious.

Note: Transcend, meaning *to go beyond limitation.*

The lightest of all bodies, the spiritual body, is closer to the truth of reality, then that of your own mind or physical body. Your spirit, *our spirits*, interpret the true essence of all life. So, it is the *perception of spirit* that shows us the *truth* in reality.

To Be, or to Become that is the question

Everyone goes through a state of Becoming. So, naturally, you follow that urge, thinking you will soon *earn* the right to just Be; which is true when concerned with your physical body, but you have to discover all your states of Being, in order to experience them…know them, and improve them.

Meditation sheds light on your path to fulfillment within, and helps one evolve their perception into one of a limitless spiritual reality…leading to a state of "Being", in all your bodies. With all this truth staring you in the face, you can't help but to shed your dense weight of negative thought, and your constant struggle to Become. You will feel the relaxed sensation of deep silence, pure awareness, and serenity, in a state of "Being"…in the *real* reality.

What is meditation?

The first thing that pops into most people's heads when they think of what meditation means to them, (if they have never experienced it), is forcing oneself to concentrate on a specific thought, and then making all thoughts disappear. Not true; yes, you may experience inner quietness, but not by forcing it to happen. Practicing TM promotes positive, lasting change in physical, mental, and spiritual health.

General Guidelines for Meditation

Put any assumptions aside, and don't worry about doing it perfect. There is no one right way of meditating. Just as every person perceives things different, everyone will have a different overall experience.

There are many different ways of meditating. The most commonly known method, is directing one's attention to improve the state of consciousness. The possibilities are endless as to what you can direct your mind towards, all of which involve the senses. Meditation is about directing your attention on some focal point, but allowing your mind and spirit to work together in revealing the origin of that thought, no matter how simple. Learning to meditate can be as simple as "waking up". Your mind must be open, not forced into any mode of thought.

To begin, find a quiet, comfortable place to meditate…somewhere you won't be bothered for at least 10 to 15 minutes. Sit in a relaxed position, with your spine as straight as possible. This allows energy to rise freely up the spine, and limits obstructions. It is a very important aspect in meditation.

A general guideline to follow when meditating, is to begin with focusing on something you already know how to sense…such as an image, a word, a sound, a smell, a taste, a vibration, and all, or none of the above.

The main thing to remember is that the longer you practice, the better results you will have. One or two times a day for just 10 to 15 minutes each time, is plenty to begin with. After some practice, you may want to increase that to 20 or 30 minutes a day. It is all up to you, and since each person is different, then each person should meditate when they feel it is necessary, or desired. In order to make your meditations more effective, you shouldn't try to do it more than is necessary. True, practice makes perfect, but there is no perfect way to meditate, and each time you do it, you will experience something different. Meditation helps you find some very powerful energies within yourself, but it takes time to reach these higher states of consciousness, and best results are achieved if the steps taken are not forced. You have to be aware of these energies, feel their presence, and know how they work, before you can attempt to understand or use them to your advantage. These higher energies tend to help you clarify your emotions, and cleanse the system of impurities, by releasing stored negative energy, which allows room for a positive atmosphere within. (The atmosphere within, can be projected into your external environment... you can actually create your own reality, to an extent). The stronger your energy vibration is, the larger it will become, which inevitably increases your own personal environment. If this process is done gradually, it is more likely that you will want to continue meditating.

To help you know when the amount of time you decided to practice is up, place a timer, clock, or other alarm under your pillow (so it won't jolt/scare you out of the meditation).

To start out, you should practice meditating at different times of the day. Eventually, you will know which time of day suits your needs best. Once you know what times of day that you get the better experiences from TM, stick with it. From then on, do it at the same time every day. Regardless of what many different experiences you may have, you need to just accept them as they are.

If one works too hard at something, it can be tiring, but meditation shouldn't be. The first objective when beginning each meditation is to relax. TM exaggerates relaxation, restoring ones strength and vitality.

Note, that if you keep an open mind, a flow of progress is allowed to become more rapid, consistent, and less limited.

Benefits of TM

TM helps you:
- Learn what your true nature is, and how to use it to help yourself and others
- Acquire lasting satisfaction from within
- Achieve your goals, because you are more aware of your capabilities, and your environment
- Increase your inner strength and energy levels
- Gain wisdom
- Learn to adapt to change in environments, or situations, and resist the negative effects of stress
- Contribute to healing yourself when ill

You can either tread through empty stagnation with your eyes closed, or open your eyes, and see that nothing is completely empty or stagnant. In something good, anyone can find a drawback, or negative side effect. What tends to be more difficult for most people is to find something good in everything and everyone…every situation.

I have found that associating a negative experience with a chance to learn from it, or a way to save you from something worse, is a fairly easy way to make room for the positive side of things.

For example, when I was a teenager (which wasn't all that long ago), I had a chance to move back to my mother's hometown. I am not saying why I had to go away in the first place, but to get to the point, I was ready to go. My bags were packed; my ride was leaving the next morning. Well, not long after packing my bags, my grandmother and I decided to go into town. The town I lived in then, (and now), was several miles away from another, yet somewhat larger town. We were going to go play pool. We got about six miles closer to town, and all of the sudden, I saw a huge pair of headlights coming straight for us! There was no time to really feel or do anything, and yet it seemed as though it took forever for each second to go by.

We were in a small 2—door Subaru hatchback. The truck that hit us was very large, and the man in it didn't get much of a scratch. If one were to take one look at the aftermath of the mangled car, you would've thought it to be impossible for us to have survived. My grandmother broke nearly every bone in her body...just another one of her many unfortunate accidents. (But, I'm beginning to believe that all of her terrible accidents very well could have kept her from having to go through an even more tragic experience). Anyway, I wasn't hurt much. Just a few broken pelvic bones, a dislocated hip joint, glass in my hands, nose, face, etc. Fairly minor injuries, compared with the pain that my grandmother must have gone through.

Now, this may seem to have no silver lining what so ever, but I'm getting to that. I had to stay where I was after getting out of the hospital. Some of it had to do with legality reasons (so we could attempt to sue the you know what out of this guy), some of it had to do with not being able to walk...it proved to be too difficult to really go anywhere or do anything else but stay and recover...but I would have to say the main reason I stayed, was because grandma and I needed each other. I needed her strength, and she needed my leg. Not that I mean she tore my leg off so she could have it...she needed me to use it to hobble around fetching food and water and whatnot...and so I could steal the remote from her and force her to watch my soaps. (She never let us watch them when we were kids). My cousin and I would watch them, and would take the remote so grandma couldn't change the channel. She couldn't move hardly any part of her body anyway, most of it was broken. We just figured if she couldn't do anything about it, this was our chance. Finally, we got her hooked. Now she watches it at least twice a week. Ok, ok, so you are probably still wandering what the silver lining is. Ok, here it is. If I hadn't of had my car accident, I wouldn't have met the father of my two daughters, nor would I have the daughters I do today. This had a major impact on my life. And, I'm not saying why, but if I hadn't of had the car accident, I would most likely be dead as of now.

So, the point to all of this is to open your eyes, and just know there is a reason for everything…no matter how pointless, and painful some events may seem. Things like this happen to make us stronger, to make us realize how important and unpredictable life is, to make us take a different approach in our lives, to help us learn from our mistakes…

A Need to Succeed

Have you ever wondered why (in a generally healthy state of mind) once you achieve something, you are satisfied for the moment, but then you always feel the need to strive for more?

Creation comes in different forms, densities, and realities. Just like the rising and the setting of the sun, from one day to the next, this wheel of movement and progress begins with light being shed on the possibilities. With potential progress, there are thoughts to judge the risk of failure. If the decision to follow your instinct is taken, there are ideas of how to succeed. At this point, you are creating the ideas in your mind, and constructing the outcome. You follow your will to finish what you have started, and once finished, you feel proud of this creative achievement. You don't stop trying once you have accomplished something, because now that you know how good it feels to be proud of yourself, (or to provide for yourself and/or others), you don't want that feeling to fade away. It is natural to follow this constant "Need to Succeed", because this is how we survive…once you eat lunch, does that mean you will never have to eat again? Of course not.

That concept alone proves that energy (spirit) is a continuous, never—ending process, that's always been there…always will be. We rely on many different forms of energy in order to survive, and we are always in need of it to keep progress in motion. Our minds and physical bodies are just in denser forms than that of the spirit.

When you plant an apple tree, what fruit do you expect to come from that tree? Well, duh…apples. So, when you plant (conceive) the thought of an apple, you might have the idea to plant an apple tree. After your tree (idea) has grown, you would harvest the apples. You might leave some of the apples on the tree, for all of those who helped you pick them. Now, you taste the apple, and feel total success, because you helped create it. It proves to be so much more satisfying to feel the success and fulfillment from providing the apple for your self, rather than ultimately depending on everyone else to do what you, yourself are also capable of. This fulfillment has come from you; the knowledge and experience will last more than a lifetime.

If you can learn to provide your own needs, and receive your own energy without depleting others, you will be in a better position to teach others how to do the same. It is good to learn from others, as it is good to share the knowledge in which you have received. As the saying goes…"If you give a man a fish, he will eat for the moment, but if you teach a man to fish, he will eat for a lifetime"…(or something like that).

More Benefits of Learning and Practicing TM

You will learn how to free yourself from the fascination with desires, by following the path of your true nature. Of course, there will still be outside influence by others, but that is where the influence will remain. For, you will know how to recognize the fact that these desires originated on the outside, rather than within you. As for the desires that *do* come from within, you will know whether they are worthy of carrying out, or just plain selfish.

Steps and Examples of Meditation

Awareness From Within

To become aware of nothing but the knowledge of essence and awareness itself, gives one the opportunity of becoming aware of their true identity through the mind's eye. Normally, the mind is more attached to the senses, and their reaction to external life. But, by practicing the following meditation, one can let their mind become more tuned in to pure awareness itself, thereby allowing the sense of the spirit to take over. (Your conscious is reconnected to the spiritual level of the mind).

1. Sit comfortably, with your eyes closed. Relax all your bodies—physical, mental (mind), and spiritual (emotional).
2. Allow your thoughts to become very quiet, yet very much alert. Detach yourself from the external, allowing outside influence to remain where it is.
3. Directing your attention inward, let your mind settle down from the active level of every day life, to a state between your conscious levels of awake and asleep.

Imagine a word, then a thought, the meaning of that thought, and the emotional energy you feel in relation to that subject. Aim the energy inward, fast enough to reach its destiny before it can be corrupted or fades by external means; yet slow enough not to jolt, or crash into yourself.

In this way, the mind is still active, but has not been forced in any one direction. Naturally, you will begin to spiritually perceive, and mentally follow the ever—growing trail of fulfillment available at the deeper levels of the mind. Eventually, your thoughts will settle down to the deepest, yet one of the highest conscious levels possible.

Balancing Yourself

Balancing yourself will help you learn how to keep your energy bodies clear, and equal with one another. It is a way to cleanse yourself of tainted interpretations of your life. The following exercises will help you to "see the glass half full…rather than half empty". It will give you the opportunity to look at the whole picture, and see the positive light within the stresses of everyday life. When you center your emotions, you see more clearly, and feel more at peace within. It allows you to see things from a third perspective.

Vertigo

Take a few minutes to visualize yourself spinning through a tunnel, (which of course would look to be smaller, the further away you look, because of our third dimensional perceptions). Quickly shut your eyes, and see nothing…just for a moment. During that moment, allow your body to feel the vibration of centrifugal force. You will probably hear the vibration as well. Open your eyes, and take one deep breath. Though this method may be effective, it should be used with caution. Some might feel dizzy afterwards.

Breath Awareness

When feeling stressed, begin to place more attention on your breathing. Gradually, take slower, fewer, and deeper breaths. When you inhale, imagine you are pulling all of your problems, negative energy, and such, inside. As you exhale, release all emotional toxins weighing heavy on your heart.

The Big Picture

Following the example above, between inhale and exhale, you can form that energy into a neutral mass. When you exhale, imagine this mass of energy as a white ball of light, rising above you, and finally descending from your head, to your toes. In this way, you can put that energy to good use. Now, you can focus on a solution, rather than the problem, and get past the now.

Healing Meditations

We all have more than one body. Primarily, these bodies are (from the most to the least dense) the physical, mental, and spiritual bodies. When one of these bodies is dissatisfied, depressed, or in a negative state of being, all bodies are affected. If not equally positive, the negative energy starts to outweigh positive energy, which eventually manifests into physical illness. "One bad apple can spoil the rest".

Example of Healing Yourself From Within

First, sit comfortably with eyes closed. Relax all your bodies as much as possible. Visualize a large ball of radiant white light moving its way from above your head, down to your toes; virtually merge yourself within the light. (To get the best results, hold the images as long as it takes not to doubt its existence/occurrence. Fully imagine each step before attempting to move this energy. Remember that if you can fully believe that what you are creating really does exist, it will.) Know that this light is medicinal, and will heal you. Have no doubt, what so ever. Know that this light will consume all toxic energies completely. The more toxic energies there are, the more powerful your medicine will be. The more negative energy the light consumes, the more positive energy will grow…

Repeat this exercise with the seven colors of the rainbow, prism, and chakras: red, orange, yellow, green, blue, indigo, and finally, violet light. When you are absolutely sure you are healed within, and feel the effect, you are done. Now, see yourself in perfect radiant health…say to yourself, "I am healed". Keep saying this to yourself until you know, beyond a shadow of a doubt, that you are healed.

(Of course, you may not feel the total effect of being healed immediately, but you will. This will at least speed up the process).

Note: If you know one of your bodies is ill, but are not sure which one, or the exact location, follow the previous example. Make sure to disperse the light evenly. If you do know where the illness/negative energy lies, simply concentrate the light to those areas. (Like the concentration of light energy through a magnifying glass, when held at the right angle in the sun.)

A Quick Healing Technique

Though physical pain/illness may result from internal suppressions, remember that the pain is outside of you. The quicker you release the negative thoughts related to sickness, the quicker you will get over it. Also, remember that every day you will feel better than the day before. This is how I got through my oral surgery…10 days without food, because I couldn't open my mouth but maybe just enough for a straw, no pain killers because they just made me sleep and vomit…I was supposed to eat with the pills, but couldn't. When I just continued saying to myself that "tomorrow I will feel better than I do today", I did even more so.

Extract Positive Energy batteries not included

- Start off like most meditations, with relaxing your bodies, and closing your eyes.
- Notice the even spreading of light and dark particles. (If you don't understand this concept, look up into the sky…not into the sun. Don't focus on anything specific. After a few seconds, you'll see what I mean). This inner screen lies between the inner and outer you.
- Focus your attention on the light particles. Imagine these particles as being absorbed within you, and the dark particles as remaining outside of yourself.
- Now, you can use this positive energy for your own benefit, or you can give it to others. If you give it away, you can always get more once you know how to acquire it.

Note: As you've probably noticed, most meditations begin with sitting in a relaxed position, closing your eyes, and relaxing all your bodies. This allows deep relaxation, lowers blood pressure, decreases stress, and relaxes the fight or flight mechanism centered in the cerebellum of the brain. Eventually, after continued practice of TM, not only are you confident within, but all your bodies will be harmonized/equalized, giving greater resistance to stress, and illness…you will have more confidence in yourself, which will help you to succeed in everything you do.

Ascension

Ascension is the ultimate goal of almost all religions or belief practices. "What is Ascension?" you may ask. Well, for starters, union with the Divine, power available with the knowledge of the collective soul and its purpose in nature...releasing one self from the limited perception of physical reality...finding unlimited and lasting satisfaction, gaining access to the higher spiritual realms...realizing and experiencing true, spiritual perception...feeling "at home" within, mental and spiritual escape from the limitations set upon mankind and the physical realms, etc.

Ascension Exercise
- Sit in a comfortable position, with your spine as straight as possible, eyes closed.
- Visualize yourself as a Being of brilliant, white light, rising above your physical body.
- Now, imagine everything around you as "Being" this light energy as well. Become One with this purifying, white, positive energy.

Dream Awareness

In order to be aware of yourself as a whole, you have to not only be able to fulfill your body, mind, and spirit, but you have to know yourself inside and out...and that includes all our bodies, even ones such as dream bodies. (There are several more bodies, than just physical, mental, and spiritual). You have to fully know what you need and desire, in order for your dreams to become a reality. Sometimes, you may realize that you had dreams and goals of doing something you never even thought you thought of. (Like, for example, me writing this book. I never really intended on publishing. It was for myself, so I could get through hard times, and always have something to look forward to...but now, I realize that if I have received knowledge, that I should likewise, share this knowledge with others as well).

We've already discussed how to physically survive, how to use transcendental meditation, among other mental exercises to clear your mind of impurities, and somewhat an example of ways to make ascension possible.

The following is a brief explanation of how to become more aware of our dreams.

1. Get ready for bed, and get comfortable.
2. Lie down, and close your eyes.
3. Think of a word and its meaning to you.
4. Tell yourself you will remember that word, thought, feeling, etc. when you wake up.
5. Direct your energy inwards, and let go.
6. Let yourself fall asleep.
7. When you wake up, you should write down the first thought, image, emotion, etc. down on paper.
8. Try this for at least a few days to a month before you decide it won't work, and take a look at the progress taking place inside while you're asleep.

You can choose a word describing a question, if you feel the need. If you repeat a word or sound slowly, and constantly during meditation, you can help keep your mind from being distracted; if done before going to sleep, you can actually make a significant impact on your subconscious impulse to create and progress, allowing for a more immediate outcome.

If you are intent upon fully believing, and knowing you will succeed in something of importance to you, try recording a word, (or several), such as "success" on a tape recorder. Repeat the word/s over and over, until the tape is over. (You will probably want to get a tape that doesn't have much recording time, otherwise, you may repeat this so many times, you might turn blue in the face, and forget the word/s). Just before retiring for the night, turn on the tape, (using a tape player that automatically switches sides will help a lot), and go to sleep. If you sleep with someone else, you may want to give him or her earplugs, use tiny earphones, or they may want to try it too. Keep doing this every night before and during sleep, even for just a few days, or until you get desired results. You might surprise yourself on how much influence you have on your subconscious mind!

Instinct relies on the subconscious mind; your inner will to achieve and succeed will answer questions you may have, resolve doubt, help you make decisions, motivate you, pave the way to success in anything, and most of all…it will give you the tools to have faith and full confidence in yourself. You will make real, what you most desire.

Even but a dream is real…what you can imagine, or conceive of, is your own will of perception. Each person has their own interpretation of what has, is, and will Become of their own reality. I think dreams play a major role in the learning of astral form and the will of its movement or existence. In a dream, you will your body to move, and it moves (or takes action) with no questions, unless fear demeans it. In a waking astral projection, you have no physical force to move your body; you have only the will, influenced mostly by the subconscious mind and past experiences. Your subconscious is influenced firstly, by the conscious mind, and secondly, by the routine of daily life. Habit creates astral form, as does fear; but when you haven't a body to return to (if your body is dead), you must will your soul to face its fear.

Astral Projection

(It might help to go take a good look in the mirror—and not just to see the physical you, but all of yourself from every perspective before trying this)

Sit or lie down comfortably, and relax completely. Visualize yourself in every aspect and detail. Now, imagine yourself sit up (you have to really feel it—you really have to feel the separation from your mundane self).

Note: If you have to, try imagining yourself roll off the side of the bed, or floating up and looking down; whatever it takes to make you feel the reality of this and really feel it with every sense and emotion of your being. Try slowly getting up and walking, flying, floating, etc. Look at your hands, your feet, go look in a mirror…

Take a Ride on the Soul Train……

If you have trouble separating your astral self from your mundane self, try tuning into a vibration of energy. Feel its presence somewhat shake your bodies away from each other. You should use all your senses while doing this. See, hear, taste, touch, smell…sense the reality of every movement, and all your discoveries.

Mantras

The more one uses their senses in the usage of thought, (such as emotions, visual perceptions, vocal rehearsal, the repeating of words, etc.), the more influence one has on the state of consciousness they are in.

The following exercise will give you an example, as to what kind of effect mantras may have, even without meditating.

- Pick a word, any word. (Something simple with 3 syllables or less).
- Repeat the word over and over, about 20—25 times. (You don't have to be fast, it isn't a tongue twister)

Eventually, the word looses its meaning, but not for long…just long enough to preoccupy the mind from thinking with your brain.

Make up a word or sound, if you want. Use whichever word or sound that produces the most beneficial effects. (Most yoga meditating experts will tell you that the words used as Mantras have to be specific…which may be the case in their type of meditating; but for now, and to begin the process, any word should do…the point is to preoccupy your mind, and keep it from wandering).

Let Go

1. Visualize yourself inside a tunnel of rings. (All these rings represent the negative experiences from your past.)

■ Now, imagine yourself going through these rings; visualize their movement in every detail, in relation to the emotional stress/energy, colors…everything.

Note: to help yourself learn to visualize this better, draw these rings (applying the vision of their associated energy) on paper. Make a bunch of these pictures, showing each action, until you've drawn the movement (basically, you're drawing a cartoon). Then, staple the pages together and flip the pictures as fast as possible with your thumb. By astrally/spiritually going through these rings, you are letting them go…leaving them behind…in the past, where they belong. Just know that they are not only in the past, but they are also now non—existent.

Possible Effects of TM

You may feel a slight shift of movement from within; as you let go of thought, you are leaving the cleansing up to your higher self. Think about how a level has a tube of water, with a bubble of air inside the water, which moves, when the level is tipped. In a sense, you are tipping your consciousness, so that the weight of your mundane world (the water) sinks below the lighter spiritual energy (air). So, when you allow your thoughts to sink to deeper levels of the mind, it allows your spiritual energy to rise above the more limited mode of thought; therefore, your spiritual perception can finally be known, and used for the more positive aims of action. (You are actually changing your modes of perception from that of the conscious, limited, physical brain, to that of the subconscious, endless "energy mind").

Sensual Techniques

You may have trouble visualizing complex ideas, but the following exercises will give you some ways to heighten your awareness, and sensing abilities.

The following exercises should help you determine which mode of perception is easier for you to use, and should also help you to develop all your senses to the best of your ability.

- Close your eyes, and *visualize* an apple.
- In your mind's eye, hold the apple. Turn it around, so you can see all aspects. *Touch* it. Feel it.
- Take a bite. Sense the *taste* of it. *Hear* the crunch.
- Feel the texture in your mouth. *Smell* it.

Try this with any object, or environment you wish. (I don't mean go out and try eating a rock, but you get the idea I hope). The more you do this, the better your sensing abilities will be. Eventually, you will be capable of using your senses with more depth and understanding than ever before.

Another thing you can try

Taste something with your nose plugged. You can see what it is, but without using the sense of smell, you can probably just barely taste it.

Walk around a familiar place, with your eyes closed. You won't see where you are going with your eyes, but you can sense things around you. After mastering this technique, try going somewhere unfamiliar. With your eyes still closed, pick up an object. What is it? Feel it with your hands. Lick/taste it. Smell it. Shake it. Does it make a sound? Once you figure out what it is, you'll notice that you can actually see it with your mind's eye.

For example, if I told you I saw a purple elephant with yellow polka—dots…chances are, that you have already imagined it. You might be surprised at how quickly your mind reacts to mental stimulation.

■ With eyes closed, have someone put several smelly things under your nose. Sniff it out. Do you know what you are smelling?

■ You can open your eyes…but now, turn on some music as loud as possible. Plug your ears. If you can still hear the music, turn it down. You may not hear the sound with your ears, but you will feel the vibration. When you can sense a vibration and sense your environment with your mind's eye, you are using spiritual perception…the sixth sense. The sixth sense is like all five of your senses in one, and yet it is its own perception.

If you loose an arm, what do you think would happen? Most likely, your other arm would become as strong as both arms put together. If you lost your eyesight, what do you think would happen? Your hearing would probably be that much more intensified. This is the concept of some of the preceding exercises.

By exercising your senses, they become stronger. After a while, you will be able to sense inner sounds, vibrations, auras, energy fields, thought projections, spiritual energy, etc. You will sense the untouchables.

Being aware of these energies raises your vibration…your energy levels…your level of consciousness… The more you practice this type of sensual stimulation, the more you will be capable of using your higher energy vibrations in every day life. This awareness gives you inner strength of will, clarity, and knowledge of how to use these energies properly. You will be capable, and more worthy of receiving knowledge from within you and your environment. You will have more control over your own successions, and you will become more receptive to the nature of spiritual consciousness/divine motives as a whole.

The more regular you are with meditation, the more permanent the results will be. Habit gives form to astral energies. Once astral form is created, it will bring itself forth...ultimately manifesting into reality.

Quick notes

- Exercise your physical body, and your body will become stronger.
- Exercise your mind, and you will expand your consciousness.
- Exercise your sensual energies, and you will become more spiritually aware of your environment.
- Balance your bodies, and you will never have reason to become ill. (Unless you don't consume natural foods, and don't provide yourself with the proper nutrition).
- Learn to love, and you will always have something to give...and "by watering others, one waters thyself."

Section 3:
Spiritual Connection Section

Knowledge

Knowledge is one of the most important and soothing gifts one can receive. There are two principle ways of learning new information:

- Personal experience
- Learning from others

One can only learn if they want to, and open themselves up to the oncoming information. Some lessons have to be learned the hard way (personal experience), but if someone weren't there to learn from trial and error, whom would we all learn from, but ourselves?

Think of how many mistakes are eliminated when everyone knows of the outcome. Think of the accomplishments man achieves, through the knowledge of experience, and handing that information down to the following generations. Where would we be without Alexander Graham Bell? Still here, but without long distance communication, (unless we had a pony express, which would make communicating much harder, and much longer), without the Internet, without cell phones…many lives are saved because of quick long distance communications, such as 911. (Though

Alexander Graham Bell was recorded in history to have been the one who invented the telephone, I hear it was first invented by some black dude who was a slave, and didn't have the means necessary to patent his idea first; so I don't want to give Bell the glory, if he didn't really invent the phone).

Where would we be, without Susan B. Anthony, who established women's voting rights so many years ago? Do you think it could have affected who has been, or will be the President of our country? Well, I'd have to say that is a given. Of course the addition of women's votes has and will always affect the outcome of who are President was, is and will be.

Everyone is different, so even if several people go through the same experience, each person will have perceived the experience in a different light. Knowing that would explain why each person might take a different route in their lives, if they learned anything at all from the experience. Each person will conceive of a different realm of knowledge…that's kind of the point.

If everyone learns something different from the same experience (earthly life), then each person can shed light on the whole of the most possible outcomes. For example, we all know from experience, that if you cut off your finger, it's going to hurt…ok, it's more realistically going to hurt like hell!! (Unless you have some serious mind over matter issues already resolved within you).

For another example, you and several other people can read the same book, but if we all had to do a book report on the book, every report will be different in one way or another. Some things will make more sense to one person than the other, certain aspects of the book will jump out at one person, as will other aspects jump out at you and not to them.

We've all been given a body, mind, and spirit. We should make the best of it…learn to fully appreciate your environment, yourself and others. Be willing to share your information, but also be open to learning knowledge from outside sources.

Destruction is Creation and yet, there stands a choice between the two

How can destruction create? Well, here's an example:

Think of a volcano. When it erupts, hot lava pours out, destroying everything in its path. But once it collides with an opposing force, (water), land is created. Here's another example:

Everyone's physical body dies…ashes to ashes, dust to dust. But the (physically) dead body decomposes, leaving more nutrients in the ground, and more growing space for other living beings. (Makes way for new life here on earth). This natural process contributes to the food chain…completes the circle of energy and life…becomes one with the energy forces.

If we never died, there would be no room to grow, and fewer, if any resources would be available. We'd all live like tuna in a can. Oh goody…like the world doesn't already have people living on top and all around each other. And besides, those who die, aren't really gone…they're just without form…without limitation…reunited with the whole of our cosmic plan.

Energy

We may have separate physical lives, as does each separate element; but eventually, we all go back to where we came from, which is of One source of energy. We will all become One at some point in our lives, and we are all connected. It is important to remember that upon the instinct to kill. We are of One source of energy. Always were, always will be. Our physical bodies are just hosts of energy…a spiritual body, inside a mental body, inside the physical body/form, part of one body of existence.

The spiritual, mental, and physical energy given/taken from the earth and its inhabitants from all living things determines its health and karmically our own. What we think and do now will forever affect us, those around us, and the earth itself.

There are many types of energy, such as (but not limited to) heat, light, radiation, electric, chemical, mechanical, mental, atomic, and nuclear. We all depend on this energy to exist, and maintain progress; and we can all fill ourselves up with this energy, any time we feel "burned out", or "low on fuel". Once one has learned how to see the beauty and feel love and appreciation for Mother Earth (and the Universe), for ourselves and others, it is not only possible to fill up on this energy, but one can also give it freely to others. "For, by watering others, one waters thy self". The universe has an unlimited supply of energy. If one can always stay in connection with universal energy, it will flow through them at higher frequencies and vibrations…it can be given freely, because once you know how to tap into this energy, more is always readily available. "There's more where that came from". (Refer to Dedication to Nana).

By the way, how is another person born into existence? Well, first by the attraction of the opposite sex (female/male). So, in my mind, cosmic, universal energy had to have been "born" out of the attraction of opposing forces, which of course collided with such great force, that the energy couldn't be stopped or contained within any single form.

Think of trying to push together two magnets, positive to positive, or vise versa. If you didn't put any pressure on the top or the bottom, the magnets would turn around, and opposing forces would pull each other together like gravity. Only, in space, there is no resistance, so gravity has that much more strength. So, when magnetic, or opposing energies turn around, they collide with great force, which creates an even more extreme amount of energy.

Once this energy is made manifest in the physical, it is too great to be sent directly to the earth, or its inhabitants, so it is refracted and radiated to us by rays…smaller increments of this energy in the form of vibrations. This concept may be better understood by imagining a lightning bolt. One single lightning bolt has massive amounts of electrical energy, but if it were to strike someone directly, most likely it would fry that person to death. But, if the energy could be refracted, one might be able to harness the energy, save it in batteries, and use it later. (That would be pretty groovy, because this amount of energy could provide massive amounts of electricity to supply the nations).

This process can also be likened to the process by which one can tap into spiritual energy, and give it purpose…direction and flow.

Our sun provides our earth and everything in it the energy needed to survive; the plants transfer sunlight into energy used for photosynthesis…a process by which the plants make food (glucose) from water, light, and carbon dioxide. Then, plant eating animals eat the plants, meat eating animals eat the plant eaters, and finally, as of now…we rule all! Well aren't we special? I'm just glad we didn't live here when the dinosaurs did! (At least not in human form).

Our sun was born out of clouds of hydrogen gas uniting with helium, which would (under the influence of gravity) break up into smaller clouds. This caused the smaller clouds to contract, and the hydrogen atoms to hurl faster and faster to the center of the gravitational pull. The clouds became so hot, they started glowing, and eventually, this caused a nuclear reaction, causing the hydrogen and helium atoms to not only unite, but to become *as* one. This caused an immense amount of energy to radiate light and heat energy outward, and the sun stopped contracting.

Now compare the process by which a star is born, with how a child is born. Woman and man unite, woman and man have hot, wild, passionate sex, (pardon me), and upon conception, child (smaller clouds) begins to form. Woman goes through agonizing pain with contractions, each coming closer and closer together. Finally, exerting what little energy is left, mother pushes child from her womb, and the child is born. Two have become one, and have passed on another ray of light/energy, and the contractions stop.

The more galaxies that form, the more space that is needed to provide room for growth, and therefore new galaxies must grow further and further away from this dimension. The further away the galaxy expands, the faster…even time speeds up. It is a continuous process that has no real beginning or end. It has been scientifically proven that the universe is "rapidly speeding up". This, along with the evolutionary concept tells me, that human consciousness is speeding up more rapidly, as a whole. It is also said that we are going through a time shift in which the planet will enter a new frequency of energy, and after the magnetic pole shift in December of 2012, that earth will enter into the fourth dimension. There are infinite dimensions in my view, but this is a huge step for humanity, and will make way for a rise in universal consciousness.

It is evident in the evolution of mankind…to have come into this world with complete fascination. A fire was once thought of as an act of God, because that generation of man could not comprehend how fire was possible. (Although, I must contradict myself in a sense, because that generation of man also had a lot longer of a life—span…so with that being said, it is very possible that man in those times had a far greater potential to realize what life was all about, due to the length of time he was given to experience life). Eventually, man would not only understand it as a universal law, but would also "replicate" and utilize this energy. Mankind as a whole has come so far in technology, scientific phenomenon, exploring outer space, and the like. Though it may seem as though man invented what exists today, we really haven't invented anything that didn't already exist in some way. We simply realized the potential for man's ability to use our resources more wisely. We have already proven the capability of directing a mouse on a computer with only the mind. (The brain, and the mind, which of course need energy to exist).

With that said, it is made obvious that every action (even thought) has its effect on the universe, and the outcome of all life. The evolution of earthly Beings, does in fact point into the same direction of flow and progress as the universe itself. And the more people who come to this point in human consciousness, especially when together, the quicker the results are when concerned with universal energies.

Here is a way to use energy to your advantage:

Create a shell of brilliant white or light blue light all around yourself and your aura. Imagine it as being a light, bright, white/blue color, like that which we perceive to be the color of the earth's atmosphere. (This light energy comes from within. You just have to let it expand all around your self). Let this personal atmosphere consume all energy it touches. (Negative and positive). The more energy consumed, the better. This will add to what energy you already possess, giving you more inner strength. Any toxic energy that is consumed can be transformed into tonic energy.

In order for energy to exist, it would have to complete a never—ending circle, with no beginning and no end. I know, you may be thinking, "if my spirit returns to where it came from, then that would mean it has to begin somewhere...therefore, that would mean that there is a beginning and an end." To answer this bluntly, there is a beginning and an end to the *stages* of life, but not in the *existence* of life/energy itself.

Chakra Energy Centers

The aura is basically the electro—magnetic field that encompasses all living beings. It can be detected and photographed with the Kirlian Photograph. Though, in a denser form, the chakras depict these energy fields, and function through the endocrine and nervous systems.

Emotions arising from within are the result of chemical reactions in the body, which would radiate vivid colors on a Kirlian photograph. The level of energy determines the luminosity of the auras/chakras in the photo. If one were to uplift themselves spiritually...emotionally, in an intense feeling of love and appreciation, and a Kirlian photograph was taken of this person's body, (particularly the chest area), the photo would graphically represent the auras/charkas/energy fields in accordance with intensity as a brilliant color of green. There would, of course be other colors showing as well, but green would be the most obvious color of energy fields shown.

The following gives reference to the chakras, and their associated colors, glands, senses, etc.

1. Root Chakra: Security, Red, Earth, Adrenal Glands, Survival, Money, Home, Sense of Smell
2. Generative Chakra: Sensation, Stimuli, Orange, Water, Gonads, Reproductive System, Sexual Organs, Food, Emotional Body, Desire, and Sense of Taste
3. Solar Plexus: Power, Yellow, Fire/Sun, Pancreas, Control/Freedom, Mental Body, Will, and Sense of Sight
4. Heart Chakra: Love, Green, Air, Blood Circulatory System, Thymus Gland (controls immune system), Partnerships, Family, Lungs, Heart, Balance, Sense of Touch
5. Throat Chakra: Cornucopia, Blue, Personal Atmosphere, Thyroid Gland, Creativity, Manifesting One's Goals, Sound/Vibration, Sense of Hearing
6. Brow Chakra: Conscious Awareness, Indigo, Pituitary Gland, ESP, 6th Sense, Spiritual Growth, Intuition, Imagination
7. Crown Chakra: Cosmic Consciousness, Violet, Pineal Gland, Brain, Nervous System, Conflict between unity and separation, Authority, Thought/Knowing

A Note About Religious Sects

Most all religions have been born long before our time, out of the fear of non—existence after death. Also, the time frame in which the most well known religious sects came about was during a time when people thought of natural disasters, fire, and the like as an act of a God (or Gods), because these concepts were unknown to them. They were right in the sense that everything existent is an act of God, but one must understand that when a volcano erupts, or a tsunami barrels into the coastline, or lightning strikes a tree…it is not because God caused it to happen solely for man's purpose. These kinds of things happen because they are inevitable…they are natural and occur on a regular basis. They are necessary to sustain life, as we know it.

Another concept to remember, (when concerned with written texts/scriptures), is that they were originally written many many years ago, being passed down from one generation to the next. Some written texts were first handed down *verbally*, from one generation to the next, and then were eventually written down. Whether the time it took to have these stories written had to do with secrecy, or illiteracy, I may never know for sure. But one thing is for sure; every person who came into contact with the stories of the past had the opportunity to re—interpret the words. And every time the stories were told, or written, or re—interpreted into another language, they were most definitely changed in one way or another. A different word here, a revision there…so we will never truly know how these scriptures started in the first place, or what their true meanings were. Each person who translates, or interprets the texts or stories, has done it with at least some minor or even major changes…just like when a rumor starts out as something relatively small, but ends up completely blown out of proportion.

Now, I am not by any means saying that these Gods and their spiritual sanctuaries don't exist. They most certainly do, but not because the God or Gods created them…they exist because with so many people fully believing they exist, and projecting their energy into that mode of thinking, man has created them from his own mind.

There are so many religions out there, and each one of them is dead—set on their beliefs; and dead—set against anyone else's that doesn't conform to theirs. In a sense, religion is like racism. Not that one belonging to a church won't accept people of a different gender, color, or ethnic background…(actually, some don't) but they won't accept people of other religions, unless they plan to change their religion.

Modes of Perception

There are five modes of perception, as most know it. These modes are:

- **Touch** (most dense mode…quite often the hardest to develop in the mind's eye.)
- **Taste** (very closely related to that of smell. The taste of something is heightened with the sense of smell, and can even be changed in your mind…for example, if you were to close your eyes, and someone let you smell some type of food, but let you taste something else that had a similar texture…most likely, whatever it was that you tasted, would taste like whatever you smelled).
- **Smell** (Closely related to that of taste).
- **Hear** (Quick mode of perception. Sound travels at 1100 feet per second, if transmitted through air…isn't very hard to develop.)
- **See** (Almost the quickest mode of perception…light, which makes visual perception possible, travels at 186,000 miles per second. With mental visualization exercises, this is not a very hard sense to develop. In fact, it is actually probably the easiest. We use our imagination/inner visualization every day, and usually without even noticing.)

Love

Every living thing needs to love and to be loved. One can never possess enough or too much compassion. Love is what created humanity (among other living beings). This world and everything in it was created out of love. One must be capable of feeling love for oneself, the universe as a whole, and everyone else.

Here's an example of how love can change hate: when someone throws hateful remarks, or energies your way, show them it didn't hurt you. Show them love, and understanding…more often than not, they will realize they were wrong for doing whatever it was that they did to you. Sometimes, they might even apologize, and open themselves up to being loved, and learning how to love others, regardless of their impurities, or opinions.

Faith

One must learn to have faith in themselves and others. Inspiration and motivation are a big part of faith. If you know someone fully believes in you (has faith in you), you are more likely to strive to be and do everything they believe you are or can be. If you just **know** you are capable of anything you strive for, you will succeed. If you can believe in the fact that the sun will rise and set, there will be a tomorrow, the seasons will come accordingly...then you already know what faith is.

The Brain, the Mind, and the Memory

The brain is limited to the facts of present reality. The mind, on the other hand, knows the course of all phases in all life, and is not limited by forces of time and space.

The brain is a record of time, space, and the knowledge learned throughout life. The mind gives meaning to those facts. The mind describes those facts through experience, sensations, emotions, etc...it is what makes the experience of memory possible. You are capable of remembering past events, and knowing the present...you are also capable of "remembering" the future.

Cosmic Energy

When you pray for wisdom, you might not receive immediate answers; they are within you, and to gain it, you must earn it (with no ulterior motives to use that knowledge for a negative purpose).

Every living thing, whether physical or spiritual makes up the Universal Spirit. We are all a face of God, and we should try to give the collective soul a good name by doing what we know is right.

For every birth of a physical life, there is a spirit chosen for it the moment it is conceived. Not that you, yourself chooses who you will be born to (if that were the case, most rich families would be enormous), but there is a reason for where you have been placed, and with who, all related to a time—frame in which you are there to achieve something (even if only a realization) of great importance to the evolution of mankind. You are born to certain parents as a way of giving you the circumstances/opportunities to achieve your own, personal purpose here on earth.

The Universal spirit is pure energy, just as in every individual spirit. In some sense or another, it has always existed, and grows every minute. The more you use that energy for good, the more that energy grows; the more you use negative energy, the more *it* grows, and the more hold it has on you.

Every branch of the Universal Spirit has a purpose, or job, if you will. The nature of the physical universe is just a replica of what exists in the vast space of the Divine; everything is as One, and yet each interpretation comes from separate bodies, just as in an ant colony. One ant is pointless. But a colony of ants…now that's a concept! We are all connected.

Creation of Evil

There is no such thing as a devil in my point of view; there is, however, such a thing as an evil willed entity created by the belief and/or practice of evil or negative actions. Fear of the existence or capabilities of evil gives energy to a formless mass of evil energy, thereby, creating evil willed entities. Since all spirits are connected, the creation of one evil willed entity could project its demonic energy into anyone's every day perceptions (sometimes without the knowledge of it being there) if you allow it...this can create havoc within, which can motivate one to make wrong choices. Credit or belief in existence creates it. Evil only exists in those who create it, believe in it, practice it, and give credit to its power. In the case of crime and punishment, as is with any other subject...knowledge is power! When one directs their attention, their personal energy towards demonic thoughts and/or actions, this holds the power, and gives it form.

Mother Earth and Father Sky

Mother Earth is like a womb of creation, much like women of the earth.

Father sky is like a bowl of regeneration, much like the men of the earth.

Mother Earth is the womb of creation, in which Father Sky impregnates with the seeds of life.

Forgive and Forget

One must always strive to forgive and forget. Yes, I know—forgetting may seem impossible, and in some cases it is. But, just because you are having a hard time forgetting about a wrong done to you, doesn't mean it's ok to force the person who wronged you to be incapable of forgetting about it. Sometimes it really seems that every time you do something good, it doesn't take long for everyone to forget about it. But when you do something wrong, it seems as though no one will ever forget. They have no trouble remembering what you've done wrong, or what they've done right. Nor does it seem that they have any trouble forgetting about what you've done right, or what they've done wrong. (Sound like a tongue twister? Get used to it. *Life* can be a tongue twister sometimes).

And, even though it may seem impossible to forget, at the very least, you should be capable of resisting the temptation to rub it in their face. And besides, we aren't born solely for the purpose of pointing out other people's faults. We all have plenty of our own imperfections to improve upon. If you expect the person you are trying to forgive, to forgive themselves and to believe they are forgiven—you can't use their past mistakes as a "Get Out of Jail Free Card" in times when you feel defensive and in the need of justifying your own mistakes. (Two wrongs don't make a right.)

And if you don't care about the person you hold the grudge against, and don't want to forgive them…that's your choice, but if that's the case— most likely, that person doesn't care if you forgive them anyway…so you're not hurting them in any way. You're only making yourself weaker, by spending your energy on them.

Karmic Energy

Absorb, give and create only positive energy (as much as possible) and you will receive only positive results. The energy you allow inside you, can become you…be careful what you allow yourself to be.

We must all consume energy to survive. We all know that. Once energy is consumed (bought, believed, allowed within), it is processed, and used. The energy is then used for another purpose. We all do this, even though we may not notice it. If we can just recognize, or at least be prepared for the oncoming energy, then it is more likely that it will be used properly, and to the best of our ability. (If you had guests coming to visit, wouldn't you prepare a place for them to sleep, and store their belongings?)

Each person carries an electrical charge. Just hold each end of a voltage meter with each hand between the index finger and the thumb. You'll see.

Depending on the apparatus you use, you will notice that your right side has a negative charge, and your left side has a positive charge. Everything you do physically is determined by electrical impulses to and from the brain. Of course, we all know that we have two brains…the right brain controls the left side of the body, and vise versa. So, if this is the case, that would mean that your right brain carries a positive charge, and your left— brain carries a negative charge. If you were to cut your left finger, and try the experiment above, the electrical output would be reversed.

There are many different types and sources of energy, but we all radiate the combination of all energies, which is the purest form of energy there is. The energy *force* is conflict between electrical charges. Think of a movie, for example. What would be the point of making a movie if there is no conflict? There is always the good guys, and the bad guys. To have a story, you have to have a plot…a point, and of course, to make the story interesting, you must have conflict, before there can be any point to the story at all. Where would James Bond be without the conflict of outwitting the bad guys? Where would Batman be without conflict? How boring life would be without hurdles to learn from. And how would you learn, if you didn't have struggles to overcome? If everything and everyone was good, how would we know what bad is? If we never had night, how would one come to appreciate the sunrise, or the sunset, or the light by which we see? Yes, how boring that would be. Without conflict, life would be an easy task, by which we would never have to try, we would never learn because we would already know everything, and we wouldn't know how to appreciate anything or anyone, because we wouldn't know what it was like to have those things or people taken away from us.

Fear, Life, and Creation

The blackness between our physical and spiritual existence can be intimidating, but putting fright aside can show you the invisible. Fright does not exist without a body to protect and the mind to allow it; and at times we must...such as when one is in danger and in the need for a quick, instinctive, and strong response. We learn as a child to be aware of danger, which in turn **should** help to prepare ourselves for spiritual danger. We learn as a soul to be aware of our own presence/conscious self, and the constant need for energy to refresh and continue it. Energy never stops or dies; it only needs a place to store it, and the will to give it a direction of flow, or purpose. Progress is made possible by the feeling of being safe. With fear consuming one's personal atmosphere, it can be very difficult to continue a positive flow of energy.

Notes

- Don't think of a stumbling block as something you'll have to overcome; think of it as something you will learn from.
- Go with your gut...natural instinct...that adrenaline pumpin' through your body...the tight feeling in your stomach...the butterflies...go with your gut. The symptoms preceding the action or reaction taken, is your guide.
- Water purification herbs: Echinacea, basil, mints, and myrrh
- When the body detects an unknown disease, it fights it off and kills it (if possible)...then remembers the strategy for future use.

What bothers me is this:
Disease > Host >Defense > Remembrance
  MAN'S INTERFERENCE (immunization shots)

Disease mutates into something worse, in order to confuse the body and take over…. MAN'S INTERFERENCE

And the cycle continues…

How long will it take before MAN'S ability to create new vaccinations is over ridden by nature?

We are basically preparing ourselves to be slaughtered by diseases, which we ourselves will have created!!

- Our country spends soooo much time and money on defense…guns, weapons, bombs…killing machines, but why? Because "everybody does it". Man can't trust one another. We have to protect ourselves, but from who? Our own kind!
- The reason I choose to live in such a desolate area is because I would rather be on my own path, with few limitations or structure created by man's society.

When you live in a city, you must follow rules made by everyone else; you follow the traffic, the signs, man's society, and paths set in stone (or on metal/cement). Mother Nature is covered with roads and buildings (man made things), and we are to be blinded by our own stench. One breathes in mostly deadly toxins, waste, and fumes…one is subjected to TONS more negative influence, and the only way to protect oneself from it, is to either be a hermit, or become like everyone else as a first line of defense.

Although, being subjected to this negative influence, consuming deadly toxins, etc. on a regular basis…being capable of resisting temptation, building resistance to heavily consumed toxins can make you stronger by building up the immune systems of all your bodies.

For example: If you were never exposed to the common cold or flu, and suddenly you were…you could very likely, so they say, "catch your death". If you were used to colds, you would get over it with comparable ease.

Obviously, there are many contradictions you may notice throughout this book…throughout life.

This struggle of opposing forces creates an environment for motivation, change, action, and a direction of flow for energy to move into.

■ Man is creating a very unhealthy environment to live in…but why? So they can profit from others being harmed or even killed. For example: We make all these candy bars, and fast food joints, wonder pills, drugs, etc. for others to consume, and then turn around and make a profit by selling the fat consumers diet substitutions, diet plans, liposuction…and for what? Because society says it looks good, it feels good…it tastes good…you're only worth something if you can provide money…you can only have money if you go against your beliefs, and live a fast paced life, making yourself a slave to money, just to survive in a man—made society. And what do we get out of all of this? A lucrative business. How? Because the people eat chemicals and pesticides, so the doctors and dentists can have a big house, a butler, and a limo…and we can make ourselves slaves to them, in order to pay them for their "good deeds".

Cigarette companies make lots of money selling cancer sticks to us, knowing we will be back…it's one of the many addictive products allowed on the market, and yet it is as addictive as heroin…only it's legal. Did you know most store—bought cigarettes contain over 100 toxic substances, such as formaldehyde, anti—freeze, chlorine, etc.? Do you know how expensive it is to buy products claiming to help you quit smoking? (Sure…let's just take the real properties away from tobacco, make the most addictive cigarettes possible by pumping them full of pesticides and fake nicotine, and then, once we catch our prey, we'll steal what little money they have left, so they can quit. If they don't quit, more money for us…we'll just devour their bodies as well).

■ I would much rather be a leader than a follower…set my own path…take my own road, which can be followed in either direction…no one ways here…no thank you, I'll make my own roads.

■ Why do we place limits on ourselves? Because we are *taught* to.

We created many, numerous laws (limits). It's our own fault we aren't truly free. "We the People" are the ones making and voting for these laws, and Presidents to rule us. What? Aren't we realistically, fully capable of ruling ourselves? Are we helpless? Or lazy? What do you think would happen if none of us voted for any law or President? What would our rulers do without us? Rule themselves? If it weren't for the "small folk", there would be no stability, or foundation for them to stand upon. The "small folk" are who puts food on their table. If money had no worth in man's society, what would the rich folks do for food, or shelter, or medicine? Surely, their lives are valuable enough to them to work for their own survival…some might be too proud to do anything for themselves. Who do you think they would come to in their time of need? The poor folk. Those who have seen hard times know how to survive. If everyone went by just one rule…just one. Everything else would fall into place. "Do unto others, as you would have others do unto you".

Success

Take a look around. What do you see? Everything we know of, as to be real, has come from a mind…all of mind as One, holding the powerful creative forces of belief in an ideal, universal reality. All that has manifested before us was first a thought, then an idea, a belief, a goal, and a projection carried out by the action of will and determination.

The mind has, does, and will continue to create the subjects of its wanders.

When one always strives to improve, tomorrow is even better than today!!

ABOUT THE AUTHOR

The compilation of these works of mine have accumulated in the dusty dark realms of drawers for several years, until finally, I ran out of room and wanted to save what seemed important to me. I have been writing off and on, and even now, I don't think my heart will ever be content with what I've learned so far from past and present experiences. My objective is to learn something new every day for the rest of my life…and in my point of view, I have a lot of life left to live, and I plan to live it to the best of my ability. Mental stimulation brings me happiness…I like to spread it around.

This book isn't based on any religion, because I don't think any one religion is the right way. The Practice of Belief, and the knowledge from experience eventually finds its own way home.

I have been writing, well…since I could write. Putting thoughts into words, and writing or typing it all down seems to have a peaceful influence upon me. I am happy to know, that my thoughts will last forever.

BIBLIOGRAPHY

TM..Discovering Inner Energy and Overcoming Stress by Harold H. Bloomfield, M.D., Michael Peter Cain, and Dennis T. Jaffe. ©1975. Published by Delacorte Press/New York.

Healing With Herbs by Michael Castleman. ©1991. Published by Rodale Press.

The Complete Soap Maker by Norma Coney. ©1996. Published by Sterling Publishing Company, Inc.

Using Plants for Healing by Nelson Coon. ©1963 (Hearthside Press) and 1979 (Rodale Press).

Nutrition Almanac by Lavon J. Dunne. ©1973, 1975, 1979, 1984, and 1990. Published by McGraw—Hill Publishing Company.

Back to Eden by Jethro Kloss. ©1972—1974, 1981—1983, 1985, 1988, and 1992. Published by Back to Eden Publishing Co.

The Soap Book by Sandy Maine. ©1995. Published by Interweave Press, Inc.

www.meditationcenter.com by Jim Malloy. ©1998

Encyclopedia of Organic Gardening by the staff of Organic Gardening and Farming Magazine. ©January, 1977. Published by Rodale Press.

Producing Your Own Power by Carol Stoner. ©1974. Published by Rodale Press.